Tasting the Magic from A-Z

The Best Food and Beverages at Walt Disney World

Trisha Daab

Illustrations by Samantha Daab

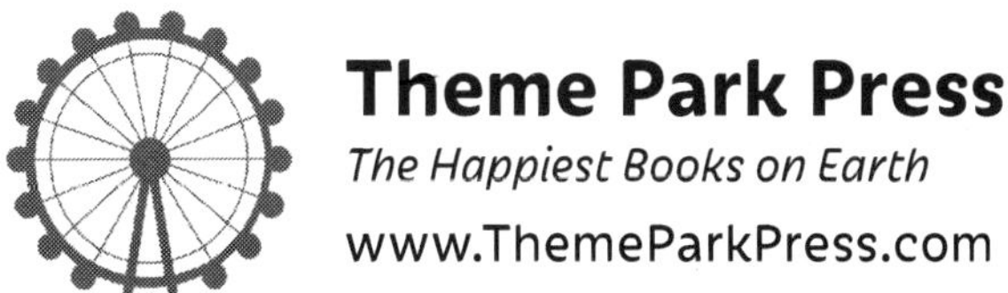

Editor: Bob McLain
Layout: Artisanal Text
Cover Art & Illustrations: Samantha Daab

ISBN 978-1-68390-107-5
Printed in the United States of America

Theme Park Press | www.ThemeParkPress.com
Address queries to bob@themeparkpress.com

This book is dedicated to my best friend and my favorite person to try new flavors with, my husband Joe. Thank you for getting me to try new foods and always being willing to travel for food, whether to Montreal or Magic Kingdom. And thanks for never judging my need for fast food tacos after a gourmet dinner.

Contents

Introduction ix

Welcome to the World of Disney Dining 1

A
Apples, Art Smith's Homecomin', Assiette Campagnarde 17

B
Beef Brewat, Be Our Guest, Beverly Soda, Breakfast, Butter Chicken 23

C
Character Meals, Church Lady Deviled Eggs, Cinderella's Royal Table, Cookies 31

D
Dawa Bar, Dining Discounts, Dining Packages & Dessert Parties 39

E
Éclair a' l'Orange, Epcot International Festival of the Holidays 45

F
Fireworks Dessert Party, Food Studios, Fruit Burger 51

G
Gaston's Tavern, Grey Stuff, Grilled Cheese 59

H
Harissa Chicken Roll, Harambe Market 63

I

Ice Cream Bar (Mickey Shaped), Ice Cream Your Way, Inside a Disney Restaurant 67

J

Jack Skellington Candy Apple, Jiko, Journals 73

K

Kiddie Cocktails, Kona Café, Kungaloosh Beer 79

L

Large Krisy Head, Les Chefs de France, Liberty Tree Tavern 83

M

Marketplaces at Epcot International Food and Wine Festival, Mickey-shaped Foods, Mugs 89

N

Naan, Nighttime Snacks 101

O

Ocean Beach Sea Salt Caramel Sundae, Outdoor Kitchens at Epcot Interntional Flower & Garden Festival 105

P

Paddlefish, Pool Bars, Popcorn, Pretzels (Mickey Shaped) 111

Q

Queso Fundido, Quick Service 117

R

Restaurant Marrakesh, Roast Beef, Room Service 121

S

Sanaa, San Angel Inn, Sci-Fi Dine-In Theatre, Spice Road Table, Starbucks 125

T

Tacos, Tiffins, Tune-In Lounge, Tutto Gusto Wine Cellar 133

U

Unique Eats, Urban Fairy Cocktail 141

V

Victoria & Albert's, Villain Cupcake 153

W

Waffle (Mickey Shaped), The Wave, Wedding Cake, Whispering Canyon Café 159

X

Xtra-Large Margarita Flight 165

Y

Yak & Yeti, Yogurt Parfait 169

Z

Zimbabwean Soda 173

Appendix A: Dole Whip, Turkey Legs and More Ways to Taste the Magic 177

Appendix B: Disney Dining Challenge 179

Appendix C: Best of Disney Dining Lists 187

Acknowledgments 193

About the Author 197

About Theme Park Press 199

Introduction

Tasting the Magic from A-Z: The Best Food and Beverages at Walt Disney World will take you on a tasty journey through Walt Disney World. This is more than a guide to eating at Disney World, it's a celebration of the food. You will:

- Experience Walt Disney World through the taste buds of fans ages 5–58, with stories and tips on where to dine and what to eat;
- Hear from current and former Disney chefs and cast members on what magical munchies they enjoy;
- Dine with us at over 35 Walt Disney World restaurants;
- Learn about dozens of Disney foods, including how they taste, where and when to find them, and a sprinkling of storytelling pixie dust on each dish;
- Enjoy the magic (and madness) of the Disney Dining Challenge: eating one dish in Walt Disney World for each letter of the alphabet; and
- Compile a list of places to try on your next Disney trip, including romantic spots, where to go with teens, finding gluten-free dishes, and dining like a Disney foodie.

In addition, you'll get answers to food questions like:

- Where should I eat at Disney World?
- How do I enjoy the Food & Wine Festival with my kids?
- Where can I dine with giraffes meandering by?
- Who decides what food will be served at all those Epcot festivals?
- Where do cast members love to dine?
- How does a Disney wedding cake taste?

- When do I bring the kids or just have a “date night?”
- How do I get a taste of the delicious Grey Stuff?

From American style fare at Liberty Tree Tavern and 50s Prime-Tme Café, to exotic eats at Sanaa and Tiffins, plus lots of snacks in between, you’ll experience Walt Disney World in foodie style.

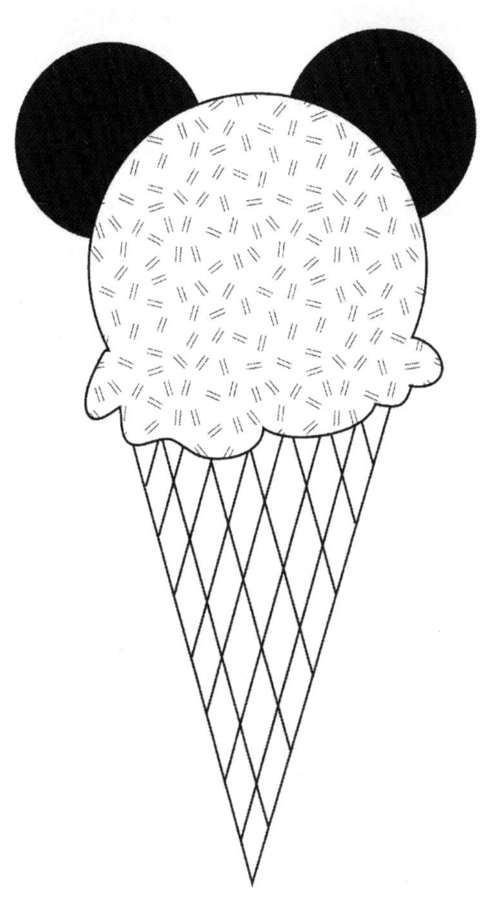

Welcome to the World of Disney Dining

Disney loves change. Whether it's modifying the tracks on Big Thunder Mountain Railroad or adding whole new lands to their theme parks, Disney World is a place where every trip brings new enchanting experiences. One area that Disney is always changing is dining. My trusty publisher and I have done all that we can to make sure all the information in this book is accurate and up to date, but just like that new-fangled cell phone morphing into the old model as soon as you walk out of the store, there will likely be a few things that Disney has decided to sprinkle with their pixie dust and change.

Mickey ice cream bars and popcorn are Disney World staples—they're not likely to go away anytime soon. But the delectable queso fundido at San Angel Inn or a favorite cocktail at Food & Wine may be on hiatus during your trip.

There are over 6,000 different types of food served at Disney World and covering them all would make this book the size of an encyclopedia. That is why you're not reading a guide, but rather a journal that includes stories, anecdotes, ideas, and even cast member and Disney chef perspectives on where you should stuff your face, and what with. So settle in, throw on your favorite Disney tunes, and maybe grab a little something to munch on, because you *will* get hungry.

300. That's an important Disney World number. Do you think it's the number of attractions? How many characters are wandering around the four parks at any given time? Maybe the number of tired kids crying on Main Street at 10pm? No, 300 is the number of places at Disney World where you can eat.

There are almost 300 different places to get your food groove on, give or take a few of those lovely Disney refurbishments I mentioned before. 300. For a food fan like yours truly, it makes me giddy. If food is not your thing, let's focus on making sure you find places that have that special Disney touch that will make your Disney vacation even more magical.

Disney World has food everywhere. You'll find it (and lots of it) at the four theme parks, at the 23 Disney resorts, at Disney Springs, and even at the water parks:

- Magic Kingdom has over 35 different eating venues, from an elegant sit-down dinner with princesses in Cinderellas Castle to a cinnamon roll the size of your head and washed down with a LeFou's Brew at Gaston's Tavern.
- Epcot, home of World Showcase and our family's vote for the dining capital of Disney World, has almost 50 options, from a palace in Morocco to under the sea at Coral Reef. And that's when there *isn't* a festival going on.
- Animal Kingdom has at least 30 ways to keep your stomach from growling. Whether it's curry dogs at Harambe Market or a Night Monkey cocktail at Tiffins, you can explore your palate's wild side.
- There are over 20 dining options at Hollywood Studios. Be transported to an old drive-in theatre for burgers and fries at Sci-Fi Dine-In or munch on pizza with the Muppets at PizzeRizzo.
- The Disney resorts have around 114 different places for you to enjoy some of the best foods and beverages, from poolside and tasty buffets, to memorable character meals.
- Disney Springs has over 46 places to grab gourmet meals and snacks.

Let's say you decided to stay at one of the gorgeous Epcot resorts: Yacht Club or Beach Club; BoardWalk Inn, or the Swan or Dolphin. From your hotel, you are only a 5–10 minute walk or a quick boat ride to 117 location options for a tasty treat. Without ever getting on a Disney bus or in a car, you can pick from the flavors of Star Wars at Hollywood Studios to a showcase of world cuisine at Epcot.

For some, that may sound like just the right variety to fill an empty stomach. For others, it will seem daunting and overwhelming. No worries. Either way, *Tasting the Magic From A-Z* has you covered.

The Disney Dining Categories

Officially, Disney has two dining categories: table service and quick service. The Disney website categorizes restaurants as one or the other. This is very important if you're on the Disney Dining Plan; and nearly as important if you're not.

At a table-service restaurant, a cast member will seat you. There are multiple types of table service:

- **FINE/SIGNATURE DINING.** Over 80 restaurants fall into this dining type, including many of the restaurants at Disney Springs, California Grill at the Contemporary Resort, Le Cellier in the Canada Pavilion at Epcot, Jiko at Animal Kingdom Lodge (AKL), and one of our new favorites, Tiffins at Animal Kingdom.
- **UNIQUE/THEMED DINING.** There is sometimes crossover between this type and character dining. These restaurants will be strongly themed in addition to having cuisine that reflects that theming, and provides a memorable dining experience. A few of our favorites are Sanaa at Kidani Village at AKL, Les Chefs de France at Epcot, Sci-Fi Dine-In at Hollywood Studios, and Whispering Canyon Café at Wilderness Lodge.
- **LOUNGES.** The place to go to grab a quick bite and an often much-needed cocktail. Tutto Gusto Wine Cellar in Italy at Epcot is our favorite lounge, with Trader Sam's Grog Grotto at the Polynesian Resort and Nomad Lounge at Animal Kingdom not far behind.
- **CASUAL DINING.** These locations offer delicious food with a bit less theming than those in the unique dining and a lower price point than fine/signature dining. Our favorite is Art Smith Homecomin' at Disney Springs.

- **CHARACTER DINING.** All character dining—from eating in the castle at Cinderella's Royal Table to hanging with Lilo & Stitch at 'Ohana—is table service.

Many, but not all, table-service restaurants will take reservations, and some require them. For very popular locations—like California Grill and Be Our Guest for dinner—a reservation may be the only way to get in.

Quick-service has two types: counter service where seating is provided and counter service where you have to find your own seat. Some quick-service locations are restaurants with ample seating like Columbia Harbour House at Magic Kingdom and Pepper Market at Coronado Springs. Others are just a truck or a stand where you order, get your food, and find the closest bench, or eat your Dole Whip while walking to the next attraction. Don't be fooled by the casualness: there are some delectable bites to be had at these locations.

How to Use This Book

This book was written as an informative, fun way to learn about some of the best food, beverages, and dining experiences at Walt Disney World. The A–Z content primarily has two type of entries:

- A food entry typically includes ordering and location tips, a description, fun anecdotes, stories, or insider information.
- A dining entry includes the location, the type of food served, and some information about or examples of the dining experience.

Additional information is provided in the appendices:

- Appendix A: Dole Whip, Turkey Legs, and More Ways to Taste the Magic
- Appendix B: Disney Dining Challenge
- Appendix C: Best of Disney Dining Lists

This book is loaded with a ton of snackable Disney World statistics about the parks, the resorts, and of course, the food.

I've pulled many of these statistics from Anthony Caselnova's *Disney by the Numbers*, also published by Theme Park Press.

Every food or dining location in this book, unless otherwise stated, was tasted by one or more members of our family ("taste testers") during a trip to Disney World, or was recommended by a Disney World cast member or chef. The taste testers range in age from 5–58 and include a range of eaters, from the adventurous to those who prefer family fare. One of us has eaten a 100-year-old egg in China; another rarely gets more exotic than a peanut-butter-and-jelly sandwich. No matter your families' taste buds, we have a taste tester with a palate similar to your own:

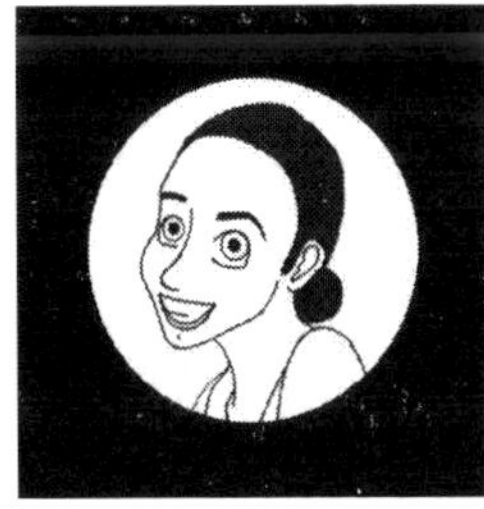

Me (Trisha), aka Mom and/or the "Not-So-Evil Stepmother." I'm not as adventurous as my husband Joe, but I love trying new things. I prefer small plates/tapas style because you get so many more options. My favorite ways to taste the magic are the butter chicken and naan at Sanaa and the lobster popcorn soup at Tiffins.

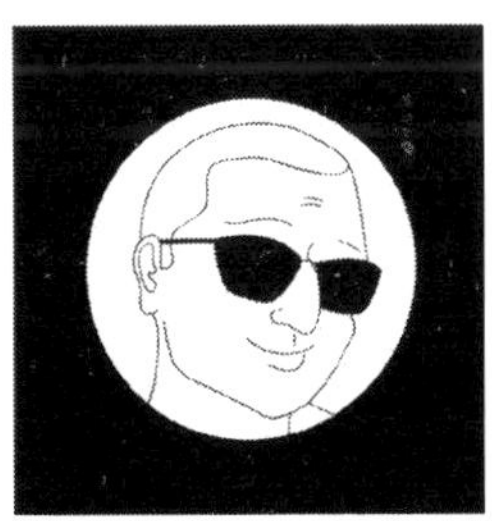

Joe, aka Dad, Bonus Dad, and my husband. Joe will eat anything, including a 100-year old egg. We always say we travel for food. He loves the salmon appetizer at Jiko and the roast beef sandwich at Be Our Guest.

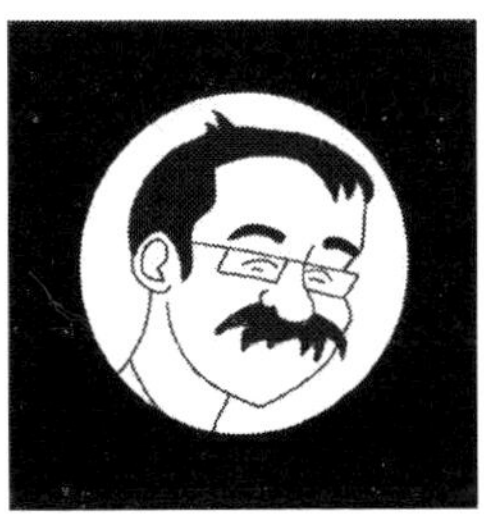

Bob, aka Bonus Dad/Stepdad and Grandpa, is a fairly adventurous eater. He will try pretty much anything once and loves seafood. "The pork shank at Jiko is my favorite food at Disney World. The risotto was creamy and the mini gourds were really good."

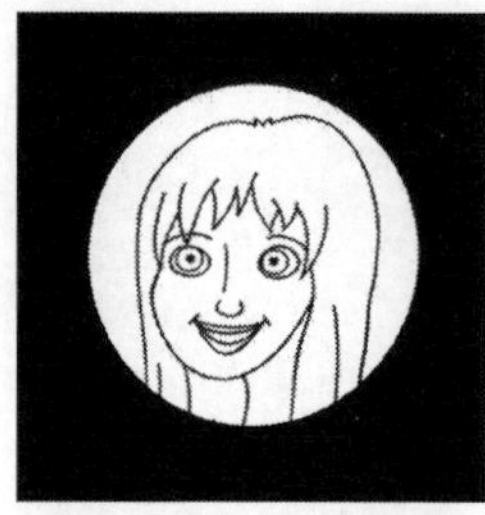

Mom, aka Debbie and Grandma, is also a fairly adventurous eater. She loves seafood, fruits, vegetables, and pie. Her most memorable Disney eats include "salmon on a plank with a hot frying pan to sear it at BOATHOUSE at Disney Springs and the yogurt parfait at Coronado Springs."

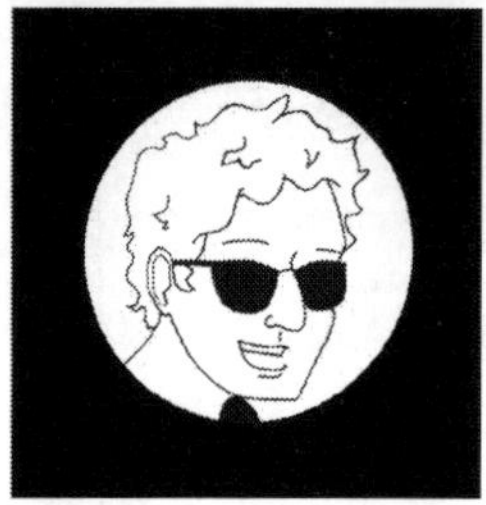

Nate, in his late twenties and recently married, had a "Disneymoon" in 2017. "The Sci-Fi Angus Burger is the best. It has bacon and apple slaw, sriracha BBQ, and pulled pork."

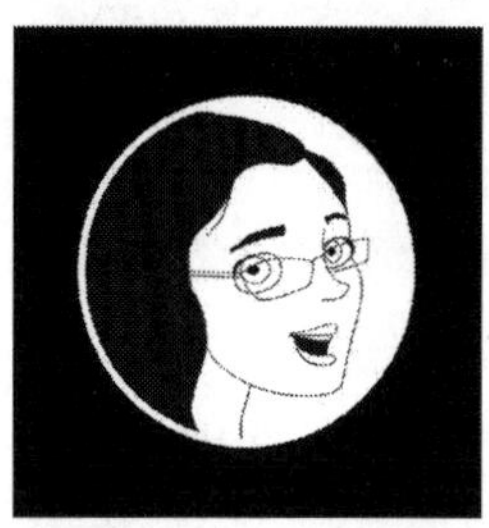

Maggie/Mags: daughter, stepdaughter, mid-twenties, avid writer, and our gluten-free expert. Salmon in salad with bacon and chili ranch is her favorite gluten-free Disney food.

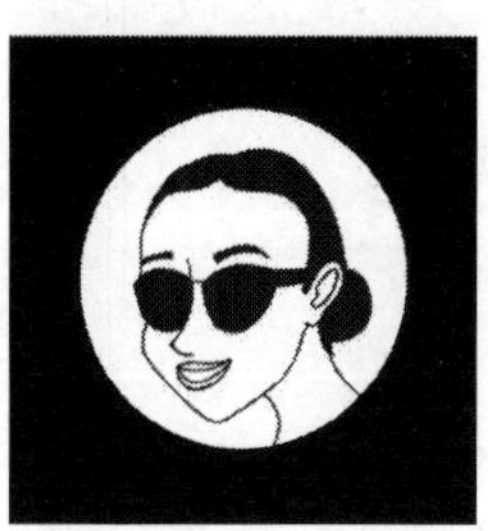

Annie/Ann: daughter, stepdaughter, college age, Tsum Tsum fanatic, and Tigger fan. Her favorite Disney food is the Mickey pretzel with cheese at Fantasmic!

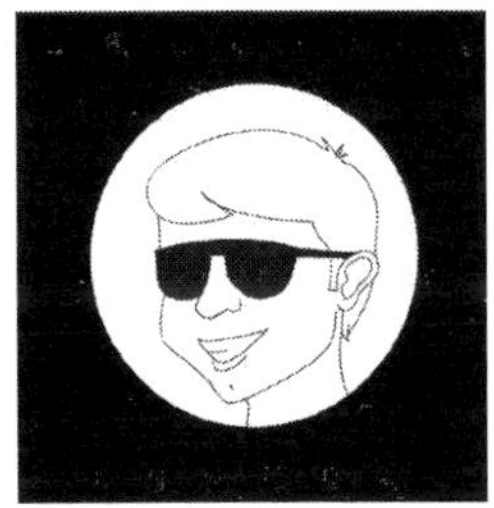

Austin/Stin: son, now a senior in high school, Disney Springs fan. "The lamb at Jiko. It was delicious."

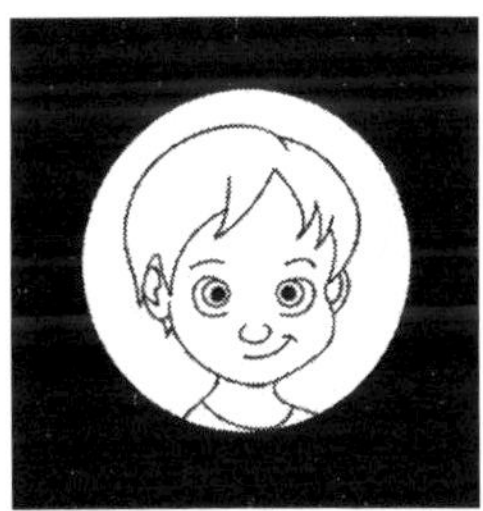

Oliver: son, young tween, resident Star Wars and superhero fanatic. "I tried some Grey Stuff and it was delicious."

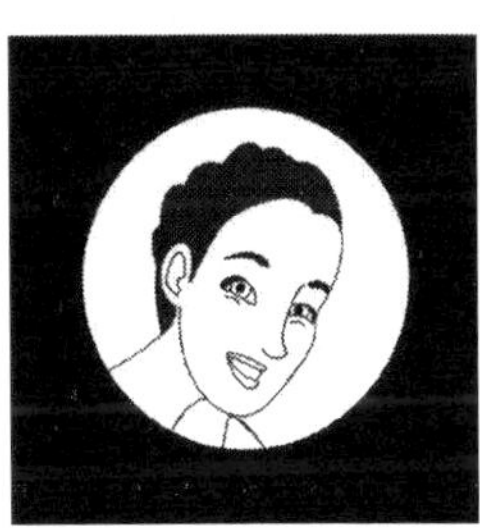

Samantha/Sam, the artist and baker of the group, and Nate's wife. "The pot de creme at Jiko. I could bathe in that."

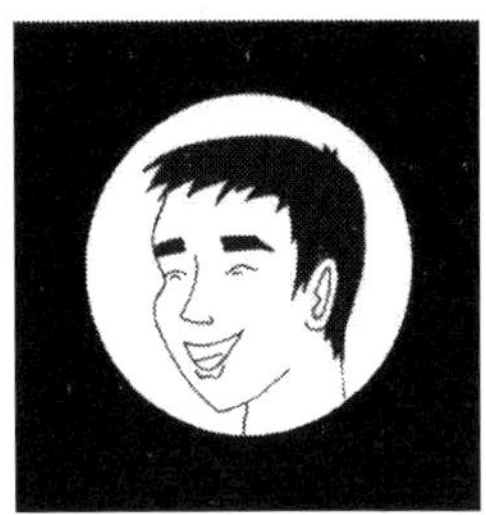

Nickolas, in his early 20s and Annie's boyfriend, challenges Oliver on being our biggest Star Wars fan. "The pork shank at Jiko. The meat was so tender it fell off the bone."

We've also enlisted the services of past and present Disney World cast members. They've worked behind the scenes in kitchens, stores, attractions, and in the offices around Disney World. They know what it's like to visit Disney as a guest, but also have the inside scoop on dining like a local.

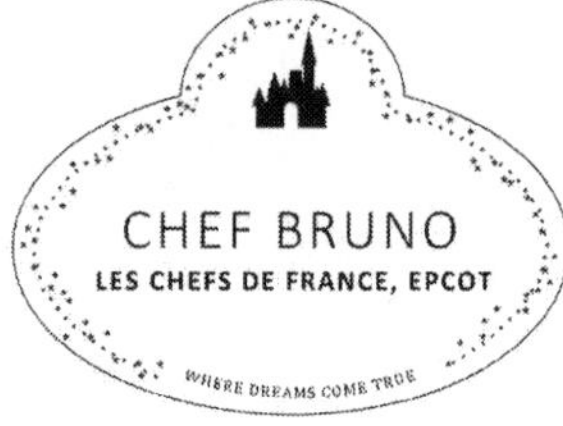

Chef Bruno is the head chef at Les Chefs de France in Epcot at the France Pavilion in World Showcase. He has been at Les Chefs for 35 years—basically since the park opened. He was hand-selected for the job by one of the original owners, famous French chef Paul Bocuse. His favorite bite at Disney World is the smoked salmon in Norway, but he says, "Les Chefs de France is the restaurant with the most beautiful view of the park. It is all right here—the people, the promenade, and the lagoon."

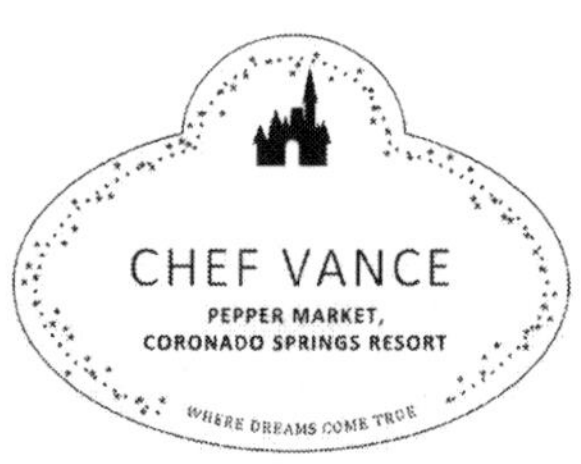

Chef Vance is a chef at Pepper Market at Coronado Springs. He has been with Disney for 8 years. Anyone who has stayed at Coronado Springs has probably seen the magical smile of Chef Vance and heard his deep, cheerful voice. He says, "The best food at Disney World is at Pepper Market. But I do like taking family and friends to California Grill at the Contemporary."

Lee was a line chef at various restaurants in Magic Kingdom, including Liberty Tree Tavern and Crystal Palace. He is now the chef and manager of operations at Elite Personal Chefs in Chicago. His favorite bite in Disney World is the falafel at Mr. Kamal's in Animal Kingdom. "I would get on a plane right now and fly to Orlando, pay to get into Animal Kingdom, eat the falafel, and just fly home to Chicago."

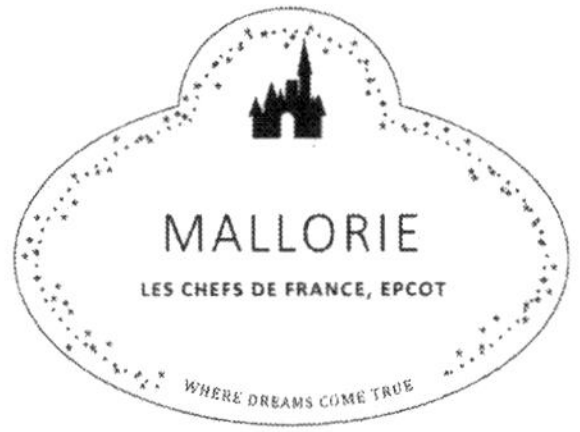

Mallorie is a team leader at Les Chefs de France in the France Pavilion at Epcot. She started her Disney career in the International College Program. "My dream was to work at Disney. Ten years after my college program was complete, the management team from France remembered me and asked for me. I came back to manage the bakery in the France Pavilion, and I now work at Les Chefs." Mallorie's favorite food in Disney World is at Les Chefs de France: "The food is really authentic. It is the food of my home."

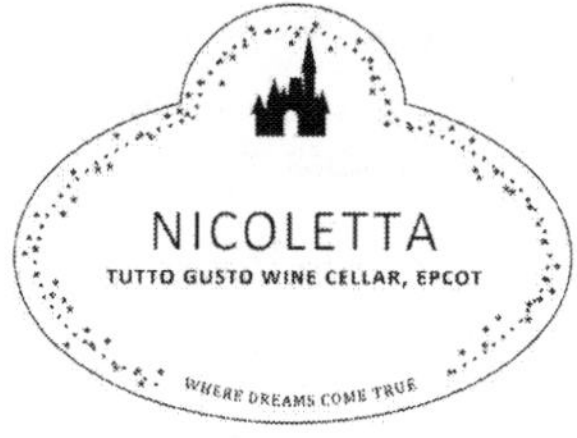

Nicoletta is a waitress at Tutto Gusto Wine Cellar in the Italy Pavilion at Epcot. She is in the International College Program and her sparkling personality is the highlight of any trip to Tutto Gusto. "Tutto Gusto is the best food in the park. I am so proud of my heritage and Italian food."

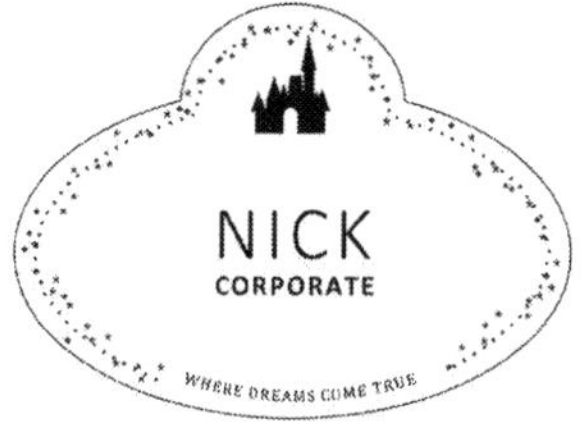

Nick works in Disney Corporate. He grew up in Florida and can remember going to Disney World as a child and watching the SpectroMagic parade. He joined the company in 2015. He loves to visit Disney World to eat and to people watch. "Half the experience for me is talking to the cast members and meeting the locals. An important part of a vacation is eating at places you've never been before and eating things you've never had. You can pick an area of the world and have food from that region at Disney World. If you time it right, you can even get food from Australia!"

Disney Dining Do's and Don'ts

DO...

- Try something new. Love all the magic you see in the attractions and shows? Disney puts it into their restaurants, too. The best and most magical restaurants at Disney are themed and offer a menu that reflects that theming. Sticking to hot dogs and burgers will mean you miss some of the most memorable experiences Disney has to offer. Also, being somewhere new may even convince that picky eater in your group to venture beyond their tried-and-true choices.
- Check online or call before leaving home because Disney constantly refreshes the magic. They call it "refurbishment." That means that the cheese fries you loved at Casey's in Magic Kingdom may no longer be available. Or your favorite cocktail at the Polynesian has some new ingredients. The food at the various Epcot festivals, special holiday treats, and fine and signature dining restaurants frequently changes in keeping with the season and the availability of the freshest ingredients. If there is something you absolutely must have, call Disney dining at 407.WDW.DINE and see if it's still available, or if they have can recommend a similar item.
- Chat with cast members when dining. Every cast member (CM) at Disney World has a story to share. Most love going to the park and have a wealth of tips and stories they are happy to share. Dining offers the perfect opportunity to have time to chat. "The CMs know what they're talking about when it comes to the food. The flavors, how to best enjoy it, they have tricks on how to eat it, what food to eat with what drink. They also have interesting stories about many of the dishes," shared cast member Nick. Chatting with the CMs around World Showcase is one of our favorite Disney pastimes. We have met a CM from France who speaks six languages, a chef who has been at

Epcot since it opened, and a lovely Italian woman whose Dad makes her pesto when he comes to visit.

- Book dining events. From sharing desserts with Stormtroopers to reserved seating at the popular nighttime shows, dining events and packages are worth it. We always book at least one each trip.
- Make dining part of the experience. Belly dancers, drive-in movies, eating in an aquarium, or dining in a castle with princesses—Disney theming and magic is not just for rides and shows. Disney realizes that eating is part of the journey and offers many ways to taste something new. Every park has restaurants that are as much about transporting you to a new place as they are about delighting your taste buds. Character meals are a must, but are only scratch the surface of what Disney has to offer. You gotta eat. Try something new while sitting in the ballroom from *Beauty and the Beast*. Eat your comfort food in a replica of a 1950s kitchen. Share some nachos under a night sky in a Mayan temple. Sample dim aum while admiring artifacts from the Himalayas or savor butter chicken as a giraffe walks by.
- Consider dining when booking your Disney resort. Disney carries the theming into every part of the hotel—from the rooms to the pools to the restaurants.
- Limit yourself to one big "experience meal" per day. If you do a character breakfast, maybe save Be Our Guest or Sci-Fi Dine-In Theater for another day. Breakfast for us is typically in the room and we try to have one character breakfast per trip. Lunch is usually the big meal of the day. We use it to take a breather and relax. This is when we have done Cinderella's Royal Table, 50's Prime Time, Les Chefs de France, or Yak & Yeti. Dinner can be a good time to try out resort restaurants. Sanaa and Jiko at Animal Kingdom Lodge are favorites because they have cuisine and dishes we've never had before. With all the different resort theming, it is an incredible opportunity to try something new and make your Disney experience even more magical by hearing the pickiest eater in your group exclaim, "I love Naan!"

- Have at least one meal a day where your whole group is together and is focused on being together, not distracted by Tigger or the trailer for *Attack of the 50 Foot Woman*. Meals are a time to connect. Talk about what you've seen, and remind yourself why you are at Disney World in the first place—to be together.
- Chef Lee insider tip on dining: check out the lunch menus at some of the fine dining table-service locations. The lunch menu will often feature items not available at dinner, and at a slightly lower price point. Lunch is also when chefs try new items. You may get a remarkable once-in-a-lifetime experience of helping create a menu at a Disney restaurant.
- Go big at lunch. If you're at Disney during the super-warm summer months, use lunch as your big meal of the day. A generous middle-of-the-day meal will get you through the many hours of sunlight ahead of you. And you will be inside an air-conditioned building during the hottest part of the day. With grandparents, college students, and kids used to eating on a set schedule, it's important to make sure everyone is getting enough to eat and drink. There are few things worse than being "hangry" in Disney World.
- On Chef Lee's must-do list: "If you are traveling with kids, go to at least one character meal. They're super fun. A lot of them are buffet-style and the buffet food at Disney is actually quite good. Everything at Disney is better than what you'd find at other theme parks. I worked at Crystal Palace for a bit and the food there was proof that buffet food can be great."
- Call Disney Dining at 407.WDW.DINE at some point during your vacation planning. Yes, it is much easier and faster to book online, but there is nothing like getting a passionate Disney cast member helping you book your dining reservations. If it weren't for the CMs at Disney Dining, I would never have learned about Whispering Canyon Café at Wilderness Lodge, watching Magic Kingdom fireworks from the beach outside the Polynesian, the exotic and delicious Sanaa at Kidani Village at AKL,

and the Fantasmic! Dinner Package. These cast members really know their Disney munchies and can even help with tips on how to get tricky reservations, like Be Our Guest at Magic Kingdom.

DON'T...

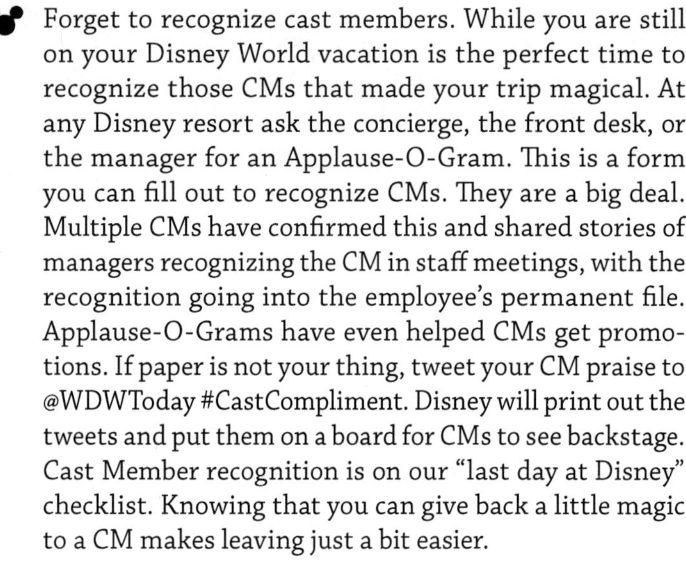

- Forget to recognize cast members. While you are still on your Disney World vacation is the perfect time to recognize those CMs that made your trip magical. At any Disney resort ask the concierge, the front desk, or the manager for an Applause-O-Gram. This is a form you can fill out to recognize CMs. They are a big deal. Multiple CMs have confirmed this and shared stories of managers recognizing the CM in staff meetings, with the recognition going into the employee's permanent file. Applause-O-Grams have even helped CMs get promotions. If paper is not your thing, tweet your CM praise to @WDWToday #CastCompliment. Disney will print out the tweets and put them on a board for CMs to see backstage. Cast Member recognition is on our "last day at Disney" checklist. Knowing that you can give back a little magic to a CM makes leaving just a bit easier.
- One of Chef Lee's dining don'ts: "A big food mistake I saw people make was not budgeting for dining or putting aside too little for dining. Open your options and get nice places on the docket. You're already at Disney, kiss your money good-bye and have some nice meals. People think they're going to go and have one nice dinner and save money on the rest of the meals, but most of the time you're not. You're going to go to some stand and walk away spending $40 on a hot dog. If it's in your budget and you want to control the amount spent on food, get the dining plan. You've saved up to go on this trip. Meals are part of the magic. So eat."
- Overschedule. Go with the flow when you can. Some of the best moments at Disney World are not planned. Make sure you have some time scheduled in each day to ask someone in your group what they want to do. One of the best parts of our 2013 trip was letting Oliver plan our days.

That meant we rode Star Tours four times in a row and took over two hours for lunch at Sci-Fi Dine-In Theater because he thought *Attack of the 50 Foot Woman* was hysterical. But it was liberating to have minimal parts of our day scheduled and to experience the magic Oliver-style.

- Miss too many meals. Sometimes your stomach needs to have more than Mickey-shaped treats, especially when you had an early start. In 2013 we left our house at 3:30am, flew to Orlando, checked into Bay Lake Tower, and then headed straight to Magic Kingdom. By 2pm we still had not had anything substantial to eat. Oliver was too excited to eat. Smart parents we are, we bought him an ice cream. And then he threw up. Another Disney first for us all! The saving grace is that he got a cute vintage Mickey t-shirt out of the deal.
- Skip breakfast. By 11am you will have used up the energy reserves from dinner the night before. Being "hangry" when you're stuck in line for Small World sweating through your second shirt of the day surrounded by overtired little girls in tiaras is not enchanting.
- Think you have to become a Disney dining expert to know where to go. Just visiting the restaurants mentioned in this book would cover you for most meals on a 7-day Disney vacation. Need more help? Call the friendly folks at Disney Dining at 407.WDW.DINE and ask an agent what they recommend.
- Schedule too many meals in one day. During our 2005 trip we had three full meals scheduled at Hollywood Studios. Late breakfast at 50's Prime Time, late lunch at Sci-Fi Dine-In, and dinner at Mama Melrose. Three sit-down meals in one day was just too much. My mom even said, "I was just too full by the end of the day. All I wanted to do was take a nap. The restaurants were all very cool. Sci-Fi Dine-In and the 50's place were almost like being in a TV show, but I could barely keep my eyes open at Fantasmic."
- Expect every moment to be perfect. Disney does all that it can to make as many moments of your trip memorable.

But sometimes there are things even Disney can't control: the weather, angry guests, long lines. As Chef Lee says, "Be Our Guest is one of the most amazing places to eat in all of Disney World. But if you're sitting next to the screaming toddler that is 3 hours past their nap, it may not seem so magical."

- Always be a member of the clean plate club. When you're sitting in a lovely air-conditioned room in a comfy chair eating a gigantic burger or a plate of spaghetti the size of Mickey's head, all that food may seem like a good idea. But when you walk out in the 90-degree heat into a crowd to wait for a parade in the Florida sun, you may regret it.
- Think every person in your party needs to order their own meal. Most of the time, Disney portion sizes are generous. If you're not a big eater or have folks in your party that can't finish a whole grilled cheese, considering sharing a plate. Most signature restaurants will split a plate for you. There may be a fee, but the fee is still less than a whole second meal that will sadly go to waste because hot dogs and pork shank aren't to-go food and don't stand a chance against the Florida heat. At quick-service restaurants, order one meal for two and ask for an extra plate so you can split it on your own. If you have a few in your group that don't like to share, don't tell them and split the food before it even gets to the table. Or if you're somewhere like Be Our Guest, send them off exploring until after the plates arrive and split the food before they come back.
- Get overwhelmed by the options. Dining can be one of the most memorable parts of any Disney vacation. There are a lot of place to eat at Disney World, but there are just as many resources to help you decide where to go. If after reading this book you still want a bit more help, give Disney dining a call at 407.WDW.DINE or find me on Facebook @authorTrishaDaab or Instagram @not-soevil_disneystepmom. I love helping folks experience Disney food magic.

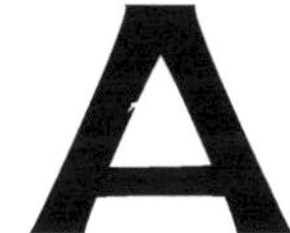

Apples

Art Smith's Homecomin'

Assiette Campagnarde

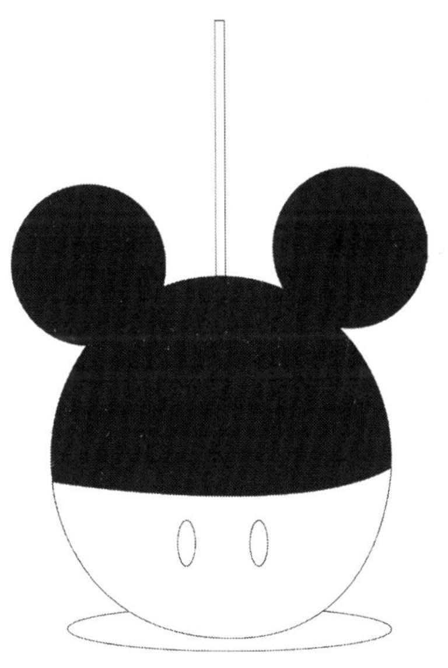

Apples

Apples are available year-round at multiple locations throughout the parks and resorts. They come in two varieties at Disney: the healthy ones we are all used to seeing and the Disney version—ginormous apples covered with a layer of caramel and sugary decorations about an inch thick.

Apple slices are featured as part of kids meals at most quick-service and table-service restaurants. Whole fresh fruit is on offer at many places throughout the parks.

But, it's in the candy-apple department where things get interesting. The apples are *huge*. If one fell out of a candy-apple tree (Disney cultivates those) and hit you on the head, you'd be out cold. The apples are colorful, and contain hundreds of grams of sugar. In fact, 741,150 pounds of sugar are used each year at Disney World, and a decent amount of it ends up on the many different varieties of candy apples.

The most famous is the classic Mickey specialty apple that can be found at Main Street Confectionery. This monstrosity is first dipped in caramel and then in milk chocolate. Then it's time for Mickey's pants, which are made by dipping the bottom of the apple in bright red sugar with two bright yellow jellybeans for the buttons. You can't have Mickey without Mickey ears. The ears are made from marshmallows. Calorie counts aren't available because you just don't want to know. And calories don't count on Main Street, right? This treat will set you back over $10, but it's very cute and quite photogenic.

Minnie is also a standard. She also starts with caramel and chocolate, but has a red sprinkles dress. The famous Minnie polka dots are done in white chocolate.

Whenever there is a new movie, event, or park attraction, special mugs and popcorn holders are sold to promote it. There will also be t-shirts, magnets, and pens a-plenty. But if you want to eat a version of your favorite character, a candy apple is the way to go. Guests munched on Nemo and Dory during the promotion of *Finding Dory* and digested Olaf during the holiday season. A candy apple makes the perfect shape for Mike from *Monsters Inc.*—covered in lime green sprinkles with a white frosting eye and bright blue sprinkles for the iris.

Location Tip: Some of the most distinctive character candy apples are sold at Main Street Confectionery in Magic Kingdom and Sweet Spells in Hollywood Studios. Goofy's Candy Company in Disney Springs lets you choose your own toppings, from Oreo cookies, Mickey sprinkles, or if you're a purist, caramel and nuts. The cutest candy-apple award goes to Zuri's Sweets Shop in Animal Kingdom. Elephant and monkey candy apples are almost too cute to eat, but they're the perfect treat for the animal lover in your group.

A visit to a Disney bakery or candy store is a must even if it's just to check out the latest candy apple creations from the Disney artists. Every season there are new and fun offerings.

Art Smith's Homecomin'

Chef Art Smith's Homecomin' is in Disney Springs, at the Landing, just a short walk from Morimoto Asia.

Homecomin' (as many cast members call it) is a taste of good ol' Southern cooking, the best Southern cooking you've ever had. Many of the dishes feature local ingredients, including some from Art Smith's own farm in Jasper, Florida.

Homecomin' has a relaxed vibe. The main dining room has exposed wood beams, comfy padded chairs, and hints of blue. The bar area has padded high-back stools and showcases rows of glasses of fresh fruit, herbs, and cocktail ingredients. There is also a walk-up bar area off a screened-in porch. Even the coasters have a sense of humor, with the names of cocktails and illustrations of bow ties, mustaches, and gingham.

It was a steamy 95 degrees when Joe and I tried Homecomin'. If it hadn't been so hot, we would have asked to be seated in the outdoor area themed like the porch of a large country home. There is also outdoor seating on the deck along the small pond in The Landing. This pond has bright Caribbean blue water with floating light fixtures. At night it's a beautiful site transforming the outdoor seating area into a romantic, softly lit, waterfront getaway. But, given the heat, we chose to eat inside.

The food and cocktails pair perfectly with the ambiance. The cocktails all feature fresh ingredients, some with Art Smith's own moonshine. The Fig and Berries Cocktail is a beautiful deep pink color with a strawberry and refreshing flavors of fig jam, fresh berries, tequila, and freshly squeezed lime. You can watch the bartender pull the ingredients for your cocktail from the row of glasses chock full of deep green herbs, large red strawberries, and bright green limes. This cocktail is refreshing and tastes like eating a juicy red strawberry straight from the vine. And the jam! All the best cocktails have jam. The fig jam adds a layer of depth and all the flavors combine and burst on your tongue.

My favorite dish was the Church Lady Deviled Eggs. We also tried the Anna Maria Fish Dip served with crisp buttermilk crackers. The dip is creamy with generous chunks of white fish. Joe preferred the fish while I savored those eggs. Both dishes are large, Disney-size portions, so we stopped ourselves at two dishes to pace ourselves for the rest of the day.

Make sure to try the Fig and Berries Cocktail, Church Lady Deviled Eggs, and the moonshine tasting. This place will change your view of moonshine with flavors like sweet tea and blue hooch.

Assiette Campagnarde

You'll find assiette campagnarde, or the charcuterie plate, at Les Chefs de France in Epcot's France Pavilion where it's available year round for lunch and dinner.

It features an assortment of different meats, mousses, and pâtés with a crusty French baguette and grainy mustard. In one plate you can sample over five different items. The offerings may change, but will typically include a creamy liver mousse, an assortment of salamis and hams, and little cornichons.

On this visit, the plate also included a complex chutney loaded with caramelized onions and sweet raisins that Joe wants to make at home. Another French staple is a rustic pâté. The pâté was chunky and had a very nutty flavor. My favorite was the salami with garlic and pepper and the chicken-liver mousse. The salami was cut into perfect bite-size circles with a touch of sweetness from the garlic and a bite from the pepper. The mousse was rich, buttery, and silky smooth. A generous smear on a crusty piece of baguette with a bit of mustard was the perfect bite.

Location Tip: Most everyone at Les Chefs is from France. The French are passionate about many things, but they are especially proud of their food. Ask your waiter or waitress about their favorite dish on the menu, their favorite wine or cocktail, or if you want some Disney news—what they think about Ratatouille finally coming to the France Pavilion at Epcot!

Les Chefs de France is one of our favorite restaurants at Disney World. From the authentic tastes of France and the bistro feel, to the passionate French cast members, this is always a must-visit while at Epcot.

During our last trip, Mallorie (a cast member from Nice, France) shared that the ham in the assiette campagnarde is her favorite. "It's the most traditional item. In France we would have the ham with cantaloupe." The flavors of this dish are so authentic that it's easy to be transported to a little French bistro on the streets of Paris. Then a sweaty guy in a Goofy hat and a fanny pack walks by and you're like, "Oh yeah. I'm at Disney World!"

B

Beef Brewat

Be Our Guest

Beverly Soda

Breakfast

Butter Chicken

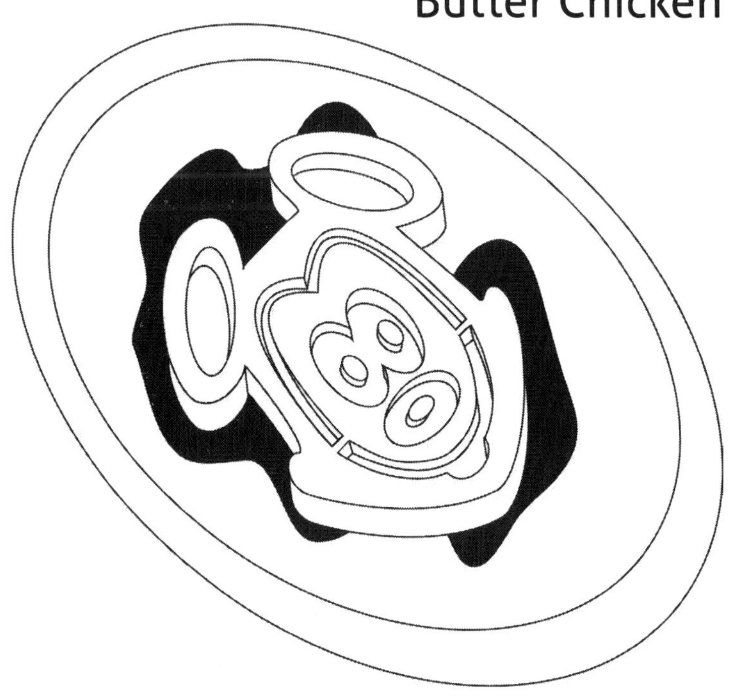

Beef Brewat

Beef brewat is served at Restaurant Marrakesh in Epcot's Morocco Pavilion where it's available as an appetizer on the lunch menu.

> **Ordering Tip**: Get more bang for you buck and try multiple exotic flavors by ordering the Combination Appetizer for Two. It includes beef brewat rolls, chicken bastilla, and a jasmina salad.

Beef brewat rolls are delicious meat pockets packed with flavor. The outside is crispy puffed pastry that is stuffed with a combination of seasoned beef and eggs. It's then sprinkled with cinnamon and sugar.

The meat on the inside is perfectly cooked and the cinnamon adds a nice bit of heat and warmth. The powdered sugar adds a melt-in-your-mouth texture, but its sweetness is balanced by the salty meat and spice of the cinnamon. The addition of cinnamon and powdered sugar may be odd to some Western diners, but using warm spices like cinnamon, nutmeg, and cardamom is common in Middle Eastern dishes.

Morocco is known for a cuisine that combines unique flavors. These flavors will make your mouth water as they perfume the air. The beef brewat rolls at Restaurant Marrakesh combine a few different traditional Moroccan dishes that are found in homes, in restaurants, and at street vendors.

Like most things in the Morocco Pavilion, the beef brewat rolls will be a new adventure for most guests—different, but not to be missed. If you want a truly magical experience that transports you to another world, Restaurant Marrakesh, with its opulent surroundings, spicy aromas, entertaining belly dancers, and a crunchy beef brewat roll, is a journey for the senses and should be on your list.

Be Our Guest

Be Our Guest is in Fantasyland at Magic Kingdom. You can hear the screams from Seven Dwarfs Mine Train during the check-in process.

It is true to the location of *Beauty and the Beast* and serves French food. At Be Our Guest (BOG), breakfast and lunch is quick service and dinner is table service. Reservations are required for all three meals. BOG is maintaining its popularity and continues to be a difficult reservation to score.

We prefer to eat here for lunch and have done so twice: in 2015 for a party of 11 and in 2016 with a party of 4. The meal begins with checking in for your reservation outside the drawbridge to the castle. After check in, the magic begins. It starts with a walk across a drawbridge where Beast's castle is peeking up over the rocks in the distance. The entrance into the castle features gargoyles and two large stained-glass double doors. The foyer is carpeted in rich reds and gold, and there is a stained-glass window of Belle and non-Beast Beast to your left, framed by heavy velvet curtains.

After waiting in a short line with rows of chatty suits of armor (listen to them, they have some interesting discussions), you go into a room with touch-screen kiosks that display a picture menu. Just touch on the food, drink, and dessert you want. If you get stuck, helpful cast members are nearby. To save time, you can also order your food in advance, but it's worth trying the touch screens at least once. Then you pay for your meal and a whole new level of magic begins.

If you don't have a MagicBand, you get a little rose that helps the server locate where you are sitting. Otherwise, your MagicBand is used. The waiters and waitresses push ornate carts with glass covers. It's all part of the theming that makes you feel as if you are at Versailles in the 18th century.

Location Tip: During dinner, Be Our Guest has a special visitor. Beast comes and walks around the dining room for autographs and pictures. If you're searching for Belle, visit the attraction next door: Enchanted Tales with Belle.

Be Our Guest has three dining rooms. The most popular, the Grand Ballroom, has pale yellow walls, an ornately painted ceiling, and large glass doors leading out onto a snowy night. During the holidays this room is even more enchanting, with garland around the balcony and a Christmas tree in front of the glass doors with snow falling gently in the background.

Another popular location is the West Wing, which is the smallest of the three dining rooms. This dimly lit room has dark ceilings and walls and the rose under a glass. The rose petals even fall. The coolest feature is a portrait of the Beast, pre-Beast. If you watch closely, you will see the portrait transform to the one from the movie with claw marks.

Location Tip: If you're looking for romance, dinner is your best bet. With red cloth napkins in the shape of roses, linen tablecloths, and non-disposable cups, the experience is more "fine dining" and less well-themed quick service. Try and get one of the small tables right up against the windows. The dark sky with the snow falling gently in the background and the soft glow of the chandeliers is a recipe for love.

In 2015, our group of 11 sat in the Castle Gallery. This room is not straight out of the movie, but has ample seating with plush booths lining the walls. The highlight of the room is a ornate statue of Beast in his regal blue suit and Belle in her stunning yellow gown dancing. It feels as if you are in a Beauty and the Beast-themed jewelry box as Belle and Beast spin to the music. The walls are covered with tapestries featuring characters in famous moments from the film. The lovely thing about this room is there is less foot traffic as you try and enjoy your meal. Go and check out the magic in the other rooms, but don't discount the Castle Gallery as a worthwhile place for a relaxing meal.

The BOG reservation technique I'm about to share will work only for breakfast and lunch as they are quick service, and your reservation is not for a specific table. It holds a space in the restaurant and you then find a table after you order. I learned this technique when trying to get 11 people into Be Our Guest during our trip in October 2015. It started with a phone call to Disney Dining and a lovely agent who said in her cheerful Disney voice, "Good luck." Her advice: be persistent. This started my regular relationship with trying to book reservations online.

One day in May it happened. I was able to get a lunch booking for 6 at 11:50am. With this renewed sense of hope I would try every day, often multiple times each day, to book online for a party of 5, then 4, then 3, then 2, and finally 1.

As October neared, additional lunch reservations started to open up and I was able to get more reservations, one person at a time. The final reservations were: 11:35 for 1, 11:45 for 1, 11:50 for 6, 11:50 for 1, 12:05 for 1 and 12:10 for 1.

Disney is smart and won't let you book multiple dining reservations under the same login. This meant I had to borrow my other family members log-ins and create new ones to book the reservations.

Now I tried to do the logical thing and contacted Disney Dining to see if they could just merge them all together. Nope. System doesn't allow that. They would have to cancel all my existing reservations and then try to re-book and there was no guarantee that the reservations wouldn't get snatched up. What the lovely agent did recommend was that we arrive all at once and the cast members at check-in would likely let us go in together. She recommended we go a few minutes before the first reservation.

She was right and the cast members were happy to let us go in together. After all that work, this place had better be amazing.

It was.

Beverly Soda

You'll find Beverly soda at Club Cool in Epcot where it's currently available year-round, but the flavors offered here do change. Beverly is a guest favorite, so it has staying power.

Ordering Tip: Beverly is free. All the sodas at Club Cool are.

Beverly is not your typical Coca-Cola flavor. It's from Italy and is used as an apertif. It is incredibly bitter, so bitter that when your friends and family are taking their first taste have the camera ready so you can capture their "Beverly Face." The reaction is priceless, like babies trying lemons.

All of our kids have tried Beverly. We have pictures of both Annie and Austin making a Beverly Face that included a crinkled nose and tongues sticking out. The flavor made me shudder, but did make me feel less full. In 2005, Nate loved trying all the flavors, even Beverly. He was very excited to keep Sam in the dark on the joy that is Beverly until after she had tried it and almost spit it out. We added a new Beverly Face to our photo collection.

Breakfast

Breakfast is an important meal of the day, but especially when at Disney World. Visiting the theme parks can be a like running a marathon. Starting the day with as much fuel as possible will help you avoid a period of "hangry" come lunchtime. There are a lot of ways to take in breakfast at Disney. Here are 5 tips to help you start your Disney day right.

- Make a quick trip to a local grocery store, convenience store, or pharmacy (Walgreens or Costco) to pick up some in-the-room breakfast items (pieces of whole fruit, juices, donuts, cereal, cereal bars, Pop Tarts). If you're using a local car service, some of them will make a stop on the way from the airport. The cost of the little boxes of cereal in the gift shops on site at Disney can bring on "sticker shock."
- Little boxes of cereal, breakfast bars, and durable fruits like bananas and oranges make a great on-the-go breakfast. They also travel well for an in-park snack.
- Schedule an early breakfast dining reservation. It's an opportunity to get in the park early and get in line for popular attractions. It's also a great time to get those awesome photos of an almost empty park. Most of the parks even have character breakfasts. If it means getting

to meet Mickey or Tigger, you may be able to get your kids out of bed even earlier.

- Grab a quick-service breakfast in the parks. There are a lot of fun restaurants that make a good breakfast spot. Every park has a Starbucks that opens early. They sell many of the standard Starbucks pastries and a few Disney-themed treats. One of our favorite breakfast spots is Gaston's in the Magic Kingdom. It is just like sitting in a scene from *Beauty and the Beast*. Plus, you can get a cinnamon roll the size of a toddler's head.
- Eat Mickey waffles! Breakfast is the time of day when you can eat the iconic Mickey waffles. Every Disney fan should try them.

Butter Chicken

You'll find butter chicken at Sanaa in Kidani Village at the Animal Kingdom Lodge where it's available year round for lunch and dinner. Sanaa is located right on the savannah. As you savor your meal, a giraffe or zebra may wander by.

Butter chicken is a total comfort food. Like comforting pot roast on a cold fall day, butter chicken is full of flavor. Sanaa serves it in beautiful clap pots with a side of basmati rice.

Kidani Village is the Disney Vacation Club Villas resort that is part of Animal Kingdom Lodge. If you're used to the Bay Lake Tower, BoardWalk or Beach Club villas, take note: Kidani Village is not in the same building as the Animal Kingdom Lodge. It's actually about a mile from the lodge. You can walk there, but if you've done enough walking that day, you can hop on a Disney bus. Just make sure to check with the driver about a stop at Kidani Village before settling into your seat.

Like most Disney restaurants, Sanaa is very accommodating to all your dietary needs, whether it's Maggie's gluten-free diet or Joe and I sharing because we had eaten too much of the bread service. In 2015, Sanaa was the pick-me-up we all needed after a 3am wake-up call and flight to Orlando. I had previously visited Sanaa when I was at Disney World for a conference. The meal and watching the animals on the savannah was so memorable that I had been looking forward to returning for over 5 years.

Joe and I shared the Potjie-Inspired. This option lets you choose two traditional African dishes with Indian overtones that are made in a sauce or gravy. Our choices were the butter chicken and spiced lamb that the server had split into separate plates as we had a sleepy Oliver sitting between us.

The butter chicken has chunks of juicy chicken that absorb the sauce, a mix of garam masala, stewed tomatoes, and cream. The sauce is a beautiful salmon color with dots of spice throughout. It's difficult to describe the flavor as it's unlike anything I've ever tasted, but it was that perfect mix of sweet and salty, with the right amount of spicy bite. Make sure to get a side of naan or save some of the naan from the bread service appetizer. Take the naan and dip it into the sauce, soaking it and you have this bite of chewy naan with the cream and spices mixing with the butteriness of the bread. It's food heaven. Using naan is much more polite than sticking your face in your bowl so as not to leave a drop of that sauce.

All nine of us had the butter chicken and loved it. Neither Nickolas nor Austin is an adventurous eater. Both of them were very skeptical of the food and ordered burgers. After some heckling and reminders that we are at Disney, where everything is delicious and you must try new things, they both took small bites and loved it. Nickolas is now the only naan and butter chicken fan in his house. Austin finally admitted liking it and even came and sat next to me so he could finish off my butter chicken and spiced lamb.

C

Character Meals
Church Lady Deviled Eggs
Cinderella's Royal Table
Cookies

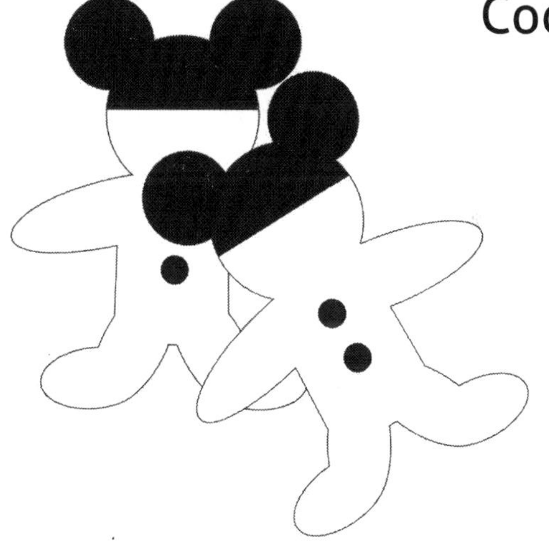

Character Meals

On every Disney trip we take with our kids, we do a character meal, typically a breakfast. There is a character meal at every park and at most of the deluxe resorts, e.g., Contemporary, Beach Club, Grand Floridian. Character meals are a must if you have a character fan in your group, and it can save you a lot of time waiting in line for autographs.

Book a character breakfast for the Fab Five (Mickey, Minnie, Donald, Goofy, and Pluto) or any characters that are must-sees on your list. Before Frozen fever and the addition of Anna and Elsa, Mickey could garner some pretty hefty lines. Annie is our characters fan; the rest of the kids were not into hanging out in a long line for a photo and an autograph. Doing a character breakfast meant Nate got his bacon, Austin his morning sugar fix, and Annie had time to give Mickey multiple hugs. Here are some of our favorite character meals:

- Crystal Palace at Magic Kingdom is home to one of the best buffets in Disney World. Find Winnie the Pooh and his friends here.
- Cinderella's Royal Table in Magic Kingdom is princess central. If you have a princess fan in your group, it is a must-do.
- Tusker House at Animal Kingdom is one of the less busy character meals featuring Mickey.

We tried Tusker House with Oliver in 2013. The characters wear khaki safari outfits, and like most character breakfasts, there are a lot of people and the dining room is big and quite loud. It's not my favorite experience, but going to an early breakfast means early admission into the park and hopping on the Kilimanjaro Safari while it's still cool enough for the animals to be more active.

Mickey waffles were a source of anticipation for Oliver as both Nate and Annie had him hyped about them. The breakfast featured a gigantic buffet with all the typical breakfast offerings, including perfectly seasoned breakfast potatoes and crispy bacon that was quite tasty when dipped in the syrup pooled around the Mickey waffle. We were lucky in that we timed our trip to the buffet perfectly and they had just brought out a new tray of Mickey waffles. The outside was crispy and the inside soft and not too sweet. Timing is also key with the blintzes. With fresh blintzes, the pastry is crisp and the inside is warm and cheesy with the sweet tartness of the cherries.

With its Animal Kingdom location, Tusker House offers a few treats—like basmati rice and sweet potato casserole—not seen at all Disney buffets. Donald greets guests outside, while the rest of the characters wander around the dining area. Each character signed Oliver's poster and gave him birthday pats on the head.

Character Meal Tip: The character meals at the resorts tend to be less busy, and many of the resorts with character meals are accessible via monorail or by walking. For example, you can escape the heat of Epcot and head over to the Bon Voyage character meal at Trattoria al Forno on the Boardwalk. Just walk over to the International Gateway at the back of World Showcase and in about 10 minutes you can be in the cool of the Italian restaurant with Ariel, Prince Eric, Rapunzel, and Finn as entertainment.

Character Meal Tip #2: Characters at the different meals can change. Make sure to call Disney Dining if you have a character on your must-see list. Lady Tremaine has been on my character list for years. Some cast members have told me that she prefers 1900 Park Fare at the Grand Floridian, but every time I've gone to book a reservation there, she is not listed among the characters. Some day the Evil Stepmother and the Not-So-Evil Stepmother will finally get to meet. And I'll ask her to autograph my Lady Tremaine Tsum Tsum. I'm sure she will just love that.

Church Lady Deviled Eggs

You'll find these little nuggets of goodness at Chef Art Smith's Homecomin' in Disney Springs where they are a standard item on the menu. Our very knowledgeable bartender said they are a staple, so a version of them probably will always be available.

Ordering Tip: These deviled eggs make a wonderful brunch food and there are six eggs in each order, giving you a healthy serving of protein for the day.

Location Tip: The full menu is served at the bar, on the covered porch, and at the outdoor seating area. For a truly Southern experience, grab a seat on the covered porch and do some people watching while enjoying moonshine and deviled eggs.

Like any respectable Southern chef, Art has mastered the art of the deviled egg. Church Lady Deviled Eggs have a classic presentation in a bright white egg holder, and are served on a bed of fresh herbs and lettuce. The filling is as light as a cloud, with tangy mustard and a salty crunch from a small piece of bacon. It's the best of breakfast foods in just one dish.

We tried the eggs two ways. Using our fingers, we picked them up and ate them whole, for an "eggs and bacon" bite. Then, with a knife and fork, we put the eggs on top of the herbs and cut them up and ate them together. You can probably guess which way we preferred! But, since we had three eggs apiece, having a little green in the Disney diet was a good thing.

Cinderella's Royal Table

Cinderella's Royal Table, in Cinderella Castle at the Magic Kingdom, offers an enchanting meal. You are dining inside Cinderella Castle, after all. The restaurant is open for breakfast, lunch, and dinner. This is a character meal, and for princess lovers, it is *the* character meal.

Characters can change, so it's worth asking when you check in who will be there for your meal. Most meals include at least three princesses, and Cinderella is always there. We have seen Ariel, Aurora, Belle, Jasmine, and Snow White. Sometimes the Fairy Godmother and Jaq and Gus may appear as well.

The meal starts by hanging out in line near some suits of armor. Before going upstairs to the restaurant, you stop and see Cinderella. She does autographs and photos in the lavishly decorated waiting area. During the holidays, this space even has a beautiful Christmas tree that Cinderella sits besides. Definitely an enchanting Christmas card photo! We have a wonderful photo of Annie in 2005 at eight years old, awe-struck at meeting Cinderella, with the lights of the Christmas tree twinkling in the background.

The food at is upscale American with eggs and French toast at breakfast. At lunch and dinner there are salads, a seared pork tenderloin, and chicken and fish options. The best part of the food is the fun names given to certain dishes. Breakfast has a Royal Children's Breakfast with eggs, bacon, and a waffle. Lunch and dinner have the Castle Salad with bacon and a poached egg or the Chef's Fish of the Day—that is, by "Cinderella's request to showcase the freshest fish in the kingdom." The most fun is had with the desserts. The Jaq & Gus is a whipped cheesecake with strawberries, and the Clock Strikes Twelve is a dark chocolate mousse with ganache and raspberry coulis. Every royal palace needs spirits, so champagnes and sparkling wines are available. Cinderella does sometimes change her mind; as a result, the menu may feature different dishes on your visit.

Reviews of the food at Cinderella's Royal Table are mixed. Some guests love it, while others find it pricey and disappointing. Compared to the food at other upscale Disney World in-park dining locations like Monsieur Paul in Epcot or Tiffins in Animal Kingdom, the food is not quite on par. But, Cinderella's' Royal Table is all about the princesses, and of course location, location, location.

Location Tip: The restaurant is on the second floor of the castle. You can choose to climb an opulent staircase or ride in a gilded elevator. Have both experiences, if possible, and do the stairs on the way in and elevator on the way out.

You can see where the restaurant is located from in the park. Go to the back of the castle and find the row of tall, ornately decorated windows. It looks as if there is a balcony that runs along the front of those windows. This is Cinderella's Royal Table. And the folks sitting by those windows inside the restaurant are now staring at you!

The dining room feels quite royal, with a high ceiling and ornate columns. The stained-glass windows each feature a coat of arms in bright reds, yellows, and royal blues. The most magical part is that you can see the rooftops of Fantasyland in the distance. It really does feel that you are in a castle with a village of small homes just outside your dining-room window.

Nate and Sam ate here on their honeymoon in 2017 and got a prime seating location at the center of the row of windows. They were able to watch as guests tested their strength at the Sword in the Stone. "We also got to have red champagne which we had never had before. It gave the place an even fancier and classier vibe," said Sam. "We were decked out in our Disney bride and groom ears and had on our Mr. and Mrs. Mickey and Minnie shirts." Every guest at Cinderella's Royal Table receives a Wishing Star. Just tell your cast member your wish and they may be able to work some Disney magic and grant it.

Cookies

Cookies are a Disney World staple. In 2013, Oliver started his first day at Magic Kingdom with a sweet sugar cookie in the shape of, and frosted to look like, Lightning McQueen. The cookie was huge, far bigger than his hand. Main Street Confectionery is common stop on the way in or out of Magic Kingdom and has some of the best cookies in Disney World.

Cookies can come in many shapes and sizes, from your favorite Disney characters to special seasonal treats. My vote for the cutest holiday cookie is the Mickey gingerbread man. It has a typical gingerbread man shape, but with chocolate Mickey ears. Bright white dots of frosting add the famous gingerbread man buttons.

Mickey's Very Merry Christmas Party (MVMCP) offers multiple holiday-themed cookies. Guests consume a whopping

300,000 cookies each night at the party. In 2016, MVMCP guests could enjoy the cookie version of cinnamon sugar toast—snickerdoodles with hot cocoa in Tomorrowland or Adventureland. Liberty Square was home to spicy ginger molasses cookies and eggnog (the kid-friendly kind). Tomorrowland had peppermint bark cookies paired with hot cocoa, and Fantasyland was host to the snowman sugar cookie with spiced apple cider or a blue snow cone. There were also gluten-free packaged cookies at each location. This party has come a long way since our last attendance in 2005 when every stop featured a sugar cookie and hot chocolate.

Zuri's Sweet Shop at Animal Kingdom is a wild place to get cookies in different animal shapes. At Epcot there are any number of places to get a delicious cookie treat. Les Halles Boulangerie in the France Pavilion has a biscuit chocolat (chocolate chip cookie). At Gelati in Italy you can get a generous helping of creamy gelato sandwiched between two chocolate chip cookies.

At most locations, including stores, there are Minnie's Bake Shop cookies. Joe and I tried one of these at Animal Kingdom after our dinner at Tiffins. Maybe it was because we had just had an incredible gourmet dinner and had spent the previous day eating our way around Epcot, but we found the cookie bland with a manufactured plastic taste. Other guests rave about them, so perhaps we just got a bad batch.

But then there are times you may just want something traditional—like Annie did, during our trip in 2005. Annie was 8 at the time and she had been keeping an open mind, trying European-style pizza in France, beef with cinnamon at Restaurant Marrakesh, and traditional African cuisine at Jiko. By the end of six days of new tastes, Annie just wanted a plain old chocolate chip cookie—not frosted like a princess head or sprinkled with Mickey confetti, just a cookie.

Now, with the My Disney Experience app, you are never more than a few clicks away from a cookie. Search on the word "cookie" in the app and you may be surprised by the number of results.

D

Dawa Bar

Dining Discounts

Dining Packages & Dessert Parties

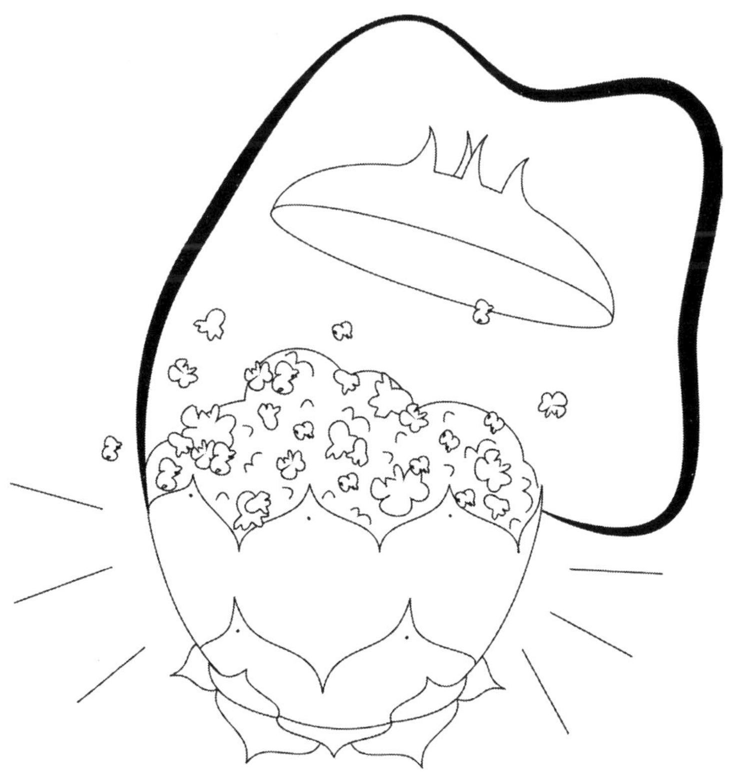

Dawa Bar

Dawa Bar is located right in front of Tusker House at Animal Kingdom, and a bit tucked back from the main drag. There is limited signage and it's easy to miss. But if you're over 21, it's worth finding.

Dawa Bar is just wine, beer and cocktails. The cocktails are delicious, but if you haven't eaten for several hours, you may want to stop by Harambe Market or the small quick-service location in front of Dawa Bar before indulging.

The venue has bar seating with fans and a canopy. With the aid of a cocktail, it's a great place to escape the heat of Animal Kingdom (which always feels like the hottest of the four parks).

Location Tip: In a hurry? Send one person over to Dawa to order the cocktails and the other to Harambe Market. Meet up at Harambe and grab a seat and enjoy some jicama and carrot slaw or curry sausage with your cocktail.

Make sure to try the Sugar Cane Mojito. It's very well made and the Dawa bartenders do larger mint leaves in place of the muddled mint. The cocktail still has all the mint flavor without the constant straw clogging that comes with mojitos of the muddled mint variety. Joe and I love a good mojito and this one does not disappoint. It's refreshing, with hints of lime, and has the right amount of sweetness from sugar-cane syrup. The drink also includes a stalk of raw sugar cane, which is fun to munch on.

Ordering Tip: The cocktail list does change. I was looking forward to trying a fruity mimosa I had read about, and the bartender informed us they no longer had it. He was as surprised as us because it was a popular cocktail.

Dining Tip: Disney chefs and mixologists never rest and are constantly experimenting with new ways to make dining magical. It's wonderful because there is always something new to try, but can be disappointing if one of your faves comes off the menu. If that happens, always ask. If they have the ingredients and the time, most cast members will help you out or will recommend dishes or drinks you may also enjoy. In this instance, the bartender recommended the mojito because, like the mimosa, it's refreshing, and has fresh flavors and fizz.

Dining Discounts

Dining is an important part of the vacation for our family. It is not the part of our Disney vacation where we tighten our purse strings, but we have found a few ways to save a bit of money on dining:

- Have breakfast in the room. Most Disney hotel rooms have a fridge, so a bowl of cereal is an option. Just be careful. Unless you are in a DVC villa room your fridge might not fit a full gallon of milk. Grab a few smaller milk cartons.
- Use the Disney Visa. It gives you 10% off at signature restaurants around Disney World. These restaurants tend to be the on the expensive side. Our Disney Visa has saved us a nice chunk of change at Jiko in Animal Kingdom Lodge, The Wave at the Contemporary, Kona Café at the Polynesian, and the Coral Reef at Epcot. You can also get 20% off at Joffrey's coffee/eat kiosks. Combining the 10% discount and the 1% back you earn on purchases can widen your Disney budget.
- Take advantage of the Disney Dining Plan, Tables in Wonderland, and free dining days.
- Bring your own food into the parks. If you don't have a car, use one of the local grocery delivery services to deliver food to your hotel. It'll be cheaper than paying Disney's prices.

Dining Packages & Dessert Parties

Is having the best seating for fireworks, parades, or shows important to you? Then check out Disney's dining packages and dessert parties.

Dining packages are a cost-effective way to get reserved seating at different shows in the four parks. These packages are different than the Disney Dining Plan, which is also sometimes called a dining packages. The dining package we are talking about here combines dining with a show that is in one of the theme parks, and requires a reservation.

Another way to get the best seats in the house is with a dessert party. A dessert party gets you reserved seating for the show and dessert, but it will put a dent in your budget.

Let's start with the cheaper option. Most dining packages give you a choice between at least two restaurants. You pick one and then reserve the time when you want to eat there. When it is time to go to your show, you're taken to reserved seating, and usually let in earlier than other guests.

Joe and I did the Rivers of Light Dining Package in 2017. Our restaurant choices were Tusker House and Tiffins. We chose Tiffins with a 4pm reservation, giving us plenty of time to brave Expedition Everest after dinner before heading to the dining package entrance for Rivers of Light at around 9pm.

At press time, the dining packages available are:

- Festival of Fantasy Parade at Magic Kingdom.
- Candlelight Processional at Epcot, a holiday-themed concert during the holiday season (mid-November through the end of December). In addition to special processional seating, you also get reserved seating for IllumiNations.
- Garden Rocks Concerts at Epcot, a seasonal event that occurs during the International Flower & Garden Festival, typically from early March to the end of May.
- Eat to the Beat Concerts at Epcot. Another seasonal event offered during the International Food & Wine Festival, typically from the end of August through mid-November.

- Fantasmic Dining Package at Hollywood Studios.
- Music of Pixar Live! Dining Package at Hollywood Studios.
- Rivers of Light at Animal Kingdom.

The kicker is that you will have a specific number of items or a pre-set menu from which you must order at the restaurant if you are not on the Disney Dining Plan. This ensures that you have more food than one person can possibly eat and that Disney gets its fair share of your dining budget.

For example, the Fantasmic Dinner Package has a pre-set menu where you choose an appetizer, entree, dessert, and drink. During our 2005 visit, the food portion of our day ended with the Fantasmic Dining Package dinner at Mama Melrose, tasty place to eat, but most of us were still full of burgers and shakes from Sci-Fi Dine-In, so we were pickey eaters that night.

Maggie, who today is gluten-free, remembers, "The pasta was amazing. I remember that pasta. Disney with gluten was just tastier." After not eating enough dinner, our group headed to a reserved seating area at Fantasmic, the park's nighttime spectacle of fireworks, lights, music, and live Disney characters.

Are the dinner packages worth it? If you don't have a full docket of rides using up your FP+ or can visit the park more than once on your trip, then try to get a same day FP+ for the show. If you're in the park during a busy time of the year, like Christmas, spring break, the summer, Thanksgiving, Festival weekends, or Friday or Saturday nights, do a dining package. You gotta eat!

Dessert parties are a bit different and will cost some extra Disney vacation dollars. Prices vary. For Joe and I to do the Fireworks Dessert Party at Magic Kingdom in 2017, the cost was $118.00. Dessert parties still have the benefit of not fighing the crowds to watch the show. These parties are becoming increasingly popular and it will only be a matter of time before there is an Animal Kingdom option. At press time, the in-park (there are out-of-park options as well) dessert party options are:

- Frozen Ever After Dessert Party at Epcot
- Happy Hallowishes Dessert Party at Magic Kingdom (during the Halloween season)
- Fireworks Dessert Party (also called Happily Ever After Dessert Party) at Magic Kingdom
- Ferrytale Fireworks: A Sparkling Dessert Cruise at Magic Kingdom
- Jingle Bell, Jingle BAM! Holiday Dessert Party at Hollywood Studios (during the Christmas season)
- Star Wars: A Galactic Spectacular Dessert Party at Hollywood Studios

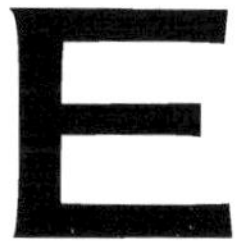

Éclair a' l'Orange

Epcot International Festival of the Holidays

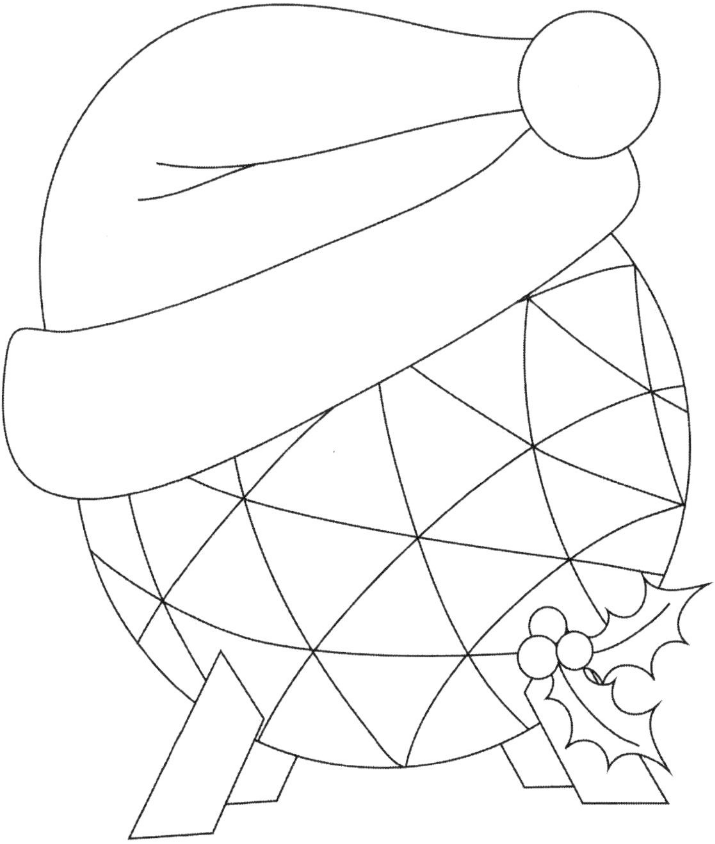

Éclair a' l'Orange

This sweet treat is served at Be Our Guest in Magic Kingdom for lunch and dinner.

The Éclair a' l'Orange is a classic French dessert. The éclair is long and thin with a crispy texture on the outside and is jammed with creamy custard filling with specks of orange zest. It's topped with a swipe of chocolate ganache, a light sprinkling of sea salt, and a thin, crunchy chocolate square with a beautiful design.

"It tastes like oranges with chocolate. It's delicious," says Austin. During our 2016 trip, that dessert was all he talked about the day we had lunch at Be Our Guest. Not being a fan of the chocolate and orange pairing, I am completely relying on Austin's love of this dessert to give you an idea of how it tastes. Hopefully these simple words are enough to tempt your palate!

Epcot International Festival of the Holidays

The holidays are one of the most magical times of year to be at Disney World. With Mickey's Very Merry Christmas Party at Magic Kingdom, all 23 resorts decked out in their festive finery, and celebrations of the traditions and food of 11 nations at Epcot, you could spend weeks and not see or taste everything. Visiting Disney World in early December is the perfect way to get into the holiday spirit. There may not be sleds or snow, but every year I'm dreaming of a Disney Christmas.

The Epcot International Festival of the Holidays is the perfect start to the season. Think of it as a scaled-down, holiday-themed version of Food & Wine—except at this festival the food kiosks are called Holiday Kitchens and there are Christmas trees everywhere.

The food at the Holiday Kitchens is like having a friend or family in that country who invites you over to join them for their holiday dinner. The dishes are a bit more "stick to the ribs" than those at the other festivals. It's a good thing it's a bit cooler in Florida this time of year.

In 2017, there are 12 Holiday Kitchens along with a quartet of Joffrey's locations serving up holiday tipples. Each Holiday Kitchen is a standalone booth, usually near the outskirts of the pavilions. But, this is the season to wander deep into each pavilion, so grab a festival treat and take a walk in a winter wonderland to see the traditional decorations from each country.

Every year Disney is adding more kitchens and more treats at each one. These are just a few of the many tastes of the holidays to try:

- Alsace Holiday Kitchen is new in 2017, and will transport you to wintertime in France with Napoléon de saumon fumé, brioche a l'aneth—a smoked salmon in a dill brioche. This is also where you will find a treat seen in bakeries around France during the holidays: buche de Noel au chocolate, a chocolate Christmas log that will be perfect with the Holiday Kir or the Spiced Rum Punch Slush. Pére Noél is coming and with all the sugary treats at the Holiday Kitchens on this list, you and your party may be on a total sugar high.
- The American Holiday Table is a taste of holiday dinner at Grandma's with slow-roasted turkey with stuffing, mashed potatoes, green beans, and cranberry sauce. Like any good home at the holidays, there are multiple wines, eggnog in grown-up and kid-friendly versions, and a cocoa candy cane with peppermint schnapps. Now if only they offered a rousing game of Monopoly that ends in a family argument, it would be truly authentic.
- Cheese fondue is on offer in the Bavaria Holiday Kitchen. The Germany Pavilion has a store filled with gorgeous *Tannenbaums* glittering with twinkle lights and handmade glass ornaments. Grab a sauerbraten with red cabbage and spåtzle, maybe paired with the glühwein (house-made spiced wine), and wander through the shops and traditional Bavarian square dripping with holiday decorations.
- Mrs. Claus and the elves have been busy at the new Cookie Nook Holiday Kitchen, baking *seven* different types of cookies and two other sugary delights. From a snowflake sugar cookie or a gingersnap cookie with cream cheese

icing and cranberry jam, to a Joy from the World Holiday Dubble brew, there are enough sweets and sips here for each one of the twelve days of Christmas.

- Feast of the Three Kings was new in 2016 and is back for 2017. The area has multiple colorful displays telling the story of when the Three Kings visit children and leave small gifts. Fresh flowers in bright blue, yellow, and lavender are everywhere. This space, and the dishes and tipples, are not to be missed. The shredded beef tamale is topped with silky smooth avocado crema and cilantro rice. Cool off with a coquito, a light coconut milk with a rum floater.
- Hokkaido Holiday Kitchen is new and offers a unique opportunity to savor the New Year, Japanese style. The New Year Celebration Soba features soba noodles with spinach in a hot soup with shrimp tempura or chicken. With KFC being a Christmas tradition in Japan, definitely give the chicken a try! Japan also has two bright red festive cocktails, the Strawberry Nigori Sake Cocktail for the grown-ups and the Iced Strawberry Milk for the kids.
- Holiday Sweets & Treats offers even more ways to need a post-holiday visit to the dentist. The peppermint sundae includes chocolate ice cream topped with whipped cream and crushed candy cane. No holiday is complete without hot chocolate, either a kid-friendly version or one for grown-ups with a choice of cordial added.
- Celebrate Feliz Navidad at Las Posadas Holiday Kitchen with Tostada de Tinga and a Horchata Margarita. The margarita tastes like a spoonful of milk and cinnamon toast crunch cereal. But with tequila. It's sweet, creamy, has a little heat from the cinnamon, and is the right kind of dangerous.
- Is a visit to the all-new Shanghai Disneyland on your wish list? At the Shanghai Holiday Kitchen sample Chinese seasonal classics like a Mongolian beef bao bun with a fortune cookie, or snack on pork and vegetable egg rolls while enjoying a mango wine.

- Buon Natale! Head to the Tuscany Holiday Kitchen for fusili di gragnano alla carbonara—pasta in a creamy parmesan sauce with pancetta and onions. Grab a panettone mignon, a miniature traditional Italian Christmas fruit cake for dessert, and wander the Italy Pavilion. The decorations are stunning and you might catch La Befana sharing her seasonal story.
- Tarabaki Holiday Kitchen in Morocco has a gorgeous selection of dishes to spice up your holiday. The highlight is the bright red and sparkling Andalusian Poinsettia Cocktail with sparkling wine, cranberry juice, and orange blossom water. A chermoula chicken drum is served with cinnamon granny apples, almonds, and brussels sprouts, and pairs beautifully with the walnut-spice coffee topped with cinnamon and whipped cream.
- The holidays in Canada taste of maple and can be found at the Yukon Holiday Kitchen and at the Canada Popcorn Cart. Pecan maple bark and a chilled maple café with brown jug maple bourbon cream liqueur are sold at the Popcorn Cart, while the Holiday Kitchen offers seared salmon with a Crown Royal whiskey glaze and a maple buche de Noel. I wonder if a toothbrush is a common gift under the tree in Canada?
- Sprinkled around World Showcase are other places to sample festive sweets and sips. United Kingdom is all about holiday tipples, such as eggnog with whiskey at the UK Beer Cart and iced Christmas toddy with Christmas tea and a cinnamon stick and Drambuie at the Tea Caddy. Make sure your wee ones don't end up on Father Christmas' naughty list and get them the Drambuie-free drink.
- In the Norway Pavilion, head to Kringla Bakeri Og Kafe for a traditional rice cream, then cool off with a snowy expedition with Elsa and Olaf on Frozen Ever After.
- Fountain View Plaza combines two favorites, Mickey and sweets, in the Mickey Santa Hat Cupcake.
- Looking for a souvenir of your magical holidays? Head to Refreshment Cool Post, home of the Mickey ornament

stein. Fill up the stein with hot cocoa and Amarula Cream or Shipyard Eggnog Porter. Pair it with the caramel-stuffed salted pretzel with soft-serve ice cream.

 Joffrey's Coffee & Tea Company Carts will keep you toasty with a Gingerbread Chai, Crazy Elf, the Warm Glow, or the Arctic Kiss Hot Chocolate.

F

Fireworks Dessert Party

Food Studios

Fruit Burger

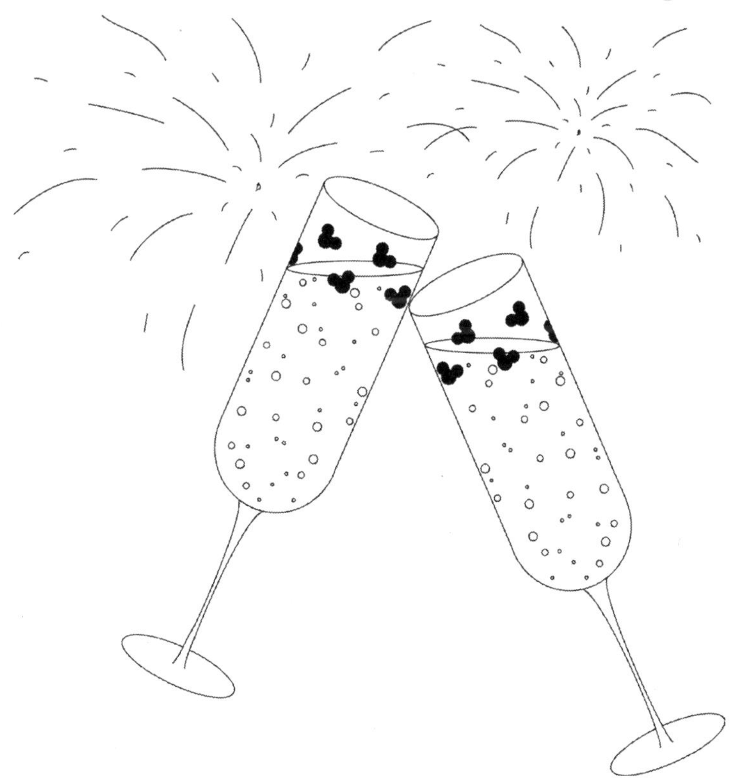

Fireworks Dessert Party

The Fireworks Dessert Party is located at Tomorrowland Terrace at the Magic Kingdom. The new nighttime show at Magic Kingdom is called Happily Ever After, so the name of this event may soon change.

To book this event, you make reservations either online or over the phone. Disney requires pre-payment for each guest. If you are at Magic Kingdom on a weekend or during one of the busy periods (spring break, summer, Halloween, Christmas), make your reservation as far in advance as possible. If there is availability, you can buy tickets at the entrance to the event, but don't count on it.

The reservation includes a dessert party that lasts for 1–2 hours, depending on when you arrive. It also includes reserved seating for the nighttime show at Magic Kingdom. For us, avoiding the gigantic crowd on Main Street and having a place to sit or stand for the show is reason enough to book this event.

Location Tip: There are two locations for this event: Tomorrowland Terrace and Plaza Garden. This determines from where you will watch the fireworks. At press time, the Tomorrowland Terrace viewing area cost a little more per ticket than Plaza Garden, likely because with Tomorrowland Terrace you have a seat and can continue munching on desserts throughout the show. Plaza Garden is the grassy area of the castle hub, in front of the Plaza Ice Cream Parlor on Main Street. You can bring a few items from the dessert party with you, but there are no desserts or drinks offered there.

When Joe and I attended the event in 2017, check-in was located at the Tomorrowland Terrace entrance closest to Main Street. A cast member gave us VIP bands providing access to the desserts and to the special seating later. A different cast member directed us to a table and gave us a quick tour of the food offerings, including the dessert buffet area, the kids desserts section (which is where the best desserts were), the "salty treats" section that includes cheese and crackers, and the drinks area.

They suggested we start heading over to the Plaza Garden viewing area about 30–45 minutes prior to the start of the show. You are supposed to ask a cast member to escort you over to the hub, but we found that you can take yourself and show your VIP band to the cast member at the Plaza Garden entrance.

There are plenty of desserts on offer at the dessert party, but it's really the special seating that drew us to this event. The drinks on offer did not include soda or anything with alcohol. We would have loved and paid a little extra to have a glass or two of Fairytale Cuvee.

Once we had our fill of the desserts we made our way over to the plaza viewing area. The hub grass is a little deceiving as it's not actually grass, but a sort of plastic alternative. Being allergic to grass, it's fine by me and is a wonderful place to get off your feet, stretch out, and even get in a little nap.

Can you sit the entire show? That depends on the crowd you're with. We had been able to sit through the show during a previous Plaza Garden viewing, but this time we weren't so lucky. We still had plenty of space and a perfect view of the new Happily Ever After show.

This new show combines all the magic of Disney fireworks with the projections on the castle and the hub grass is one of the best places to view it. It's far enough away that you can see the entire castle, but close enough that you can see details like the Hunchback of Notre Dame climbing his way to the bells. I am a huge fan of this new show and seeing it this way was well worth the expense.

If you or anyone in your group hates crowds, consider biting the bullet and booking this event. With just Joe and me, the cost was $118.00, which is a lot for good seating. We definitely wouldn't do it if we were with our whole family, as the cost would make our heads spin.

If desserts are your thing, and you want to do a stellar dessert party, head over to Hollywood Studios for Star Wars: A Galactic Spectacular Dessert Party. The desserts here are spectacular, you can meet a Star Wars character, and

Stormtroopers escort you into the party. Knowing what is on offer at Hollywood Studios, the Fireworks Dessert Party at Magic Kingdom falls short for us. There are no characters, there is little to no ambiance, and the desserts are mediocre.

Food Studios

If you've ever wondered what would happen if Andy Warhol decorated Pop Tarts or Monet crafted cocktails, the Food Studios at Epcot International Festival of the Arts are the place for you. Festival of the Arts is like being at a super-cool interactive art museum, a museum that will let you climb in paintings and serves gourmet food and drinks. Learn and create, drink a Night Sky and Paint a Cookie with a Princess in the most magical art fest on earth.

Festival of the Arts was new in 2017. Like all the Epcot festivals, food and cocktails were an important feature. "The coolest thing about Festival of the Arts is the food," shares cast member Nick. "All of the food is vibrant and there are a lot of desserts with cool confectionery art." What is the name of a food kiosk that serves artful plates and desserts? A Food Studio, of course!

"Every dish looks like art. At first you think you don't want to eat because it's so pretty," says Nick. "But you eat and drink—a lot, because it's as delicious as it is beautiful." In 2017 there were eight Food Studios with four Joffrey's Coffee and Tea Company locations serving up photo-worthy cocktails. At Festival of the Arts, the food kiosks are not always a small building on the outskirts of a pavilion as they are at Food & Wine and Flower & Garden. If you want to experience all of the artsy eats, you may have to venture into a few of the pavilion restaurants.

Festival Tip: Visit characters during the festival. Each character has a painting or drawing near them. Alice had a beautiful drawing of the White Rabbit staring anxiously at his watch. Shockingly, Belle was captured reading.

At press time, it was a bit too soon to say what the next Festival of the Arts will bring, but the first one featured:

- Artist's Table featured white scallops with chorizo and a stroke of bright red from the roasted red pepper coulis. Flights aren't just for wine here; they are for sipping chocolate that came in both little artist and boozy artist versions. The grown-up version had dark chocolate with an intense raspberry flavor from the Chambord.
- Block & Hans had festival wines and a few beer options.
- Cuisine Classique was home to the Artist Palette Jumbo Chocolate Chip Cookie. The giant, palette-shaped cookie has a hole for your hand and was served with frosting paint and a paint brush so you can channel your inner Monet. Also on the menu was a braised beef short rib with parsnip puree paired with the Campo Viego Rioja art series.
- Decadent Delights had all sweets on display. The dark chocolate s'mores had vanilla kisses and white chocolate fire. The Deconstructed Purple Sweet Potato Pie had a deep purple palette-shaped cake with dollops of marshmallow whipped cream and fresh fruit as the paints. Cherry Herring Liqueur and Courvoisier got the creative juices flowing.
- $E=AT^2$ is where art and science meet. There was a lot of "deconstruction" on this menu, like the Deconstructed BLT with crispy pork belly, tomato jam, and soft-poached egg. This studio raised the bar for the Artist Palette cookies with a Figment white chocolate painting with an edible chocolate easel, and a White Chocolate Mickey Puzzle also with an artist palette. Cocktails got the $E=AT^2$ treatment with a Deconstructed Breakfast of Apple Chai Tea Shake topped with maple bourbon cream, a waffle crisp, and candied bacon. For the kids and kids at heart there was a Pop-Artsicle that's blue, white, and red just like the popsicles from the ice cream truck.
- El Artista Hambriento (The Hungry Artist), near Mexico, was a taste of a global masterpiece. The Choriqueso Taco had chihuahua cheese and a splash of red and green

peppers. The Huarache was a flank steak with black beans, salsa de chile de arbol, chipotle mayo, and pops of color from the red cabbage, shredded carrots, and frisee lettuce.

- If you already need another Artist Palette Cookie, head to Fife & Drum.
- Funnel Cakes added some spice to this tasty dessert a gingerbread funnel cake plenty big enough to share.
- Japan served futomaki sushi at the Kabuki Café kiosk and a chirashi sushi and sashimi at Tokyo Dining.
- At the Joffrey's carts, artists scored their caffeine in concoctions like the Cinnamon Sensation, the Dreamy Bourbon, the Night Sky Latte, the Painted Lady Latte (with Baileys and whipped cream).
- Joy of Tea inspired animal artists with traditional Chinese golden fish and a panda rice cake.
- Les Halles Boulangerie-Patisserie always has pastry pieces of art on display and added an elegant opera cake to its menu for Festival of the Arts.
- Masterpiece Kitchen gave meats the sculptor treatment with the charcuterie palette. The plate had creatively arranged artisanal meats, duck breast, and cheese. Characters got ready for their close-up with the Mickey and Pluto white chocolate painting with an edible chocolate easel. Guests grabbed a classic sidecar with a chocolate twist for the trip to the next studio.
- Morocco had house-made falafel with pickled beets, turnips, and Tahini sauce
- Painter's Palette served two of the must-have festival eats: the trio of savory croissant doughnuts and Pop't Art. The doughnuts were little sandwiches that pack a powerful punch of flavor with a whipped herb cream cheese with sea salt; chicken mousse with fresh herbs; and spicy tuna with sriracha mayo and sesame seeds. The Pop't Art looks like Andy Warhol got his hands on the breakfast staple Pop Tarts. Dessert was a designed sugar cookie with chocolate hazelnut filling and colorful frosting art.

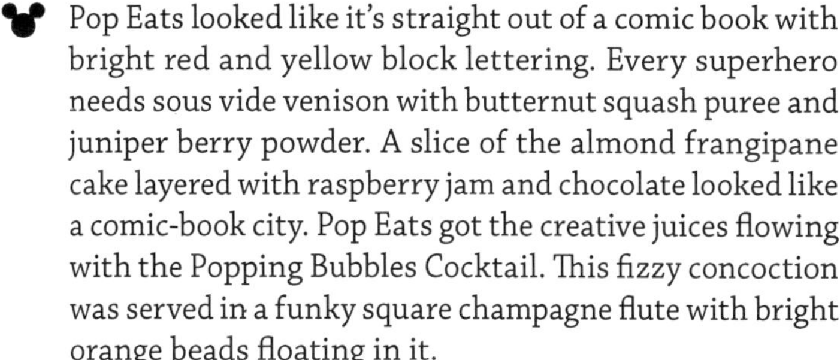

- Pop Eats looked like it's straight out of a comic book with bright red and yellow block lettering. Every superhero needs sous vide venison with butternut squash puree and juniper berry powder. A slice of the almond frangipane cake layered with raspberry jam and chocolate looked like a comic-book city. Pop Eats got the creative juices flowing with the Popping Bubbles Cocktail. This fizzy concoction was served in a funky square champagne flute with bright orange beads floating in it.
- Refreshment Cool Post had chilled shrimp, quinoa, and layered vegetables with spice yogurt and red pepper coulis. For breakfast, a sweet and colorful version of the croissant doughnut was available at Refreshment Port. It's topped with pastry cream, bright white frosting, and a variety of metallic and colored pearls.

Fruit Burger

Also known as a macaron with fresh fruit, it got the moniker "fruit burger" from Oliver during a breakfast trip in 2013. Joe and Oliver grabbed sweet treats at Les Halles Boulangerie Patisserie for breakfast while I tried a Flower & Garden Outdoor Kitchen. Oliver had a fruit tart that had multiple layers of pastry and fruit drizzled with a sugary glaze and a raspberry macaron that he decided was a fruit burger.

Enjoy your own fruit burger at Les Halles Boulangerie in Epcot's France Pavilion. Les Halles also offers a rainbow of other chic and délicieux macarons.

Ordering Tip: Les Halles is a great place for breakfast. Most of World Showcase officially opens at 11am, but Les Halles opens earlier, typically at 9am.

The fruit burger is two crispy sweet macarons that envelop a sweet cream with fresh fruit. The flavors available may change, but have included a soft red raspberry macaron with a raspberry and lime cream that is ringed by fresh raspberries. It's a beautiful, bright, fruit-burger-looking treat.

G

Gaston's Tavern

Grey Stuff

Grilled Cheese

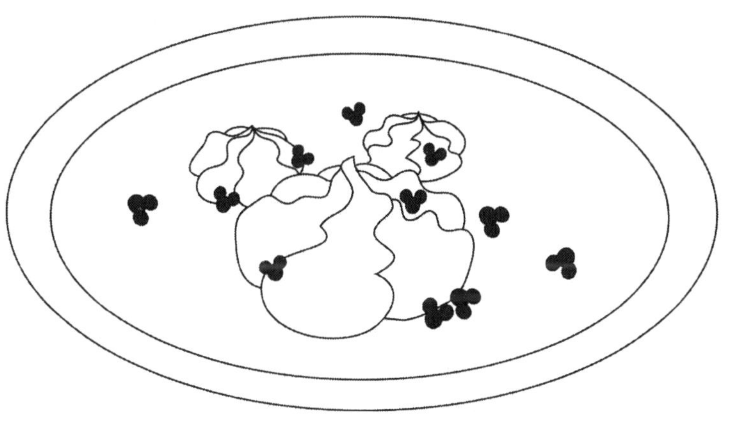

Gaston's Tavern

Gaston's Tavern is a quick-service restaurant tucked back in the French village area of Fantasyland at Magic Kingdom. It's open for breakfast, lunch, and dinner, and typically has the same menu all day. So, if you want a side of something beefy with your gigantor cinnamon roll, head to Gaston's.

Make sure to try LeFou's Brew in a souvenir cup. The drink is a super-sweet frozen apple juice with toasted marshmallow. To give a true brew look, the drink is topped with passion-fruit mango foam. Most kids will love it, some adults may find it too sweet. The best part is the cool stein or goblet it's served in.

We have this great plastic brown beer stein with an emblem of jolly LeFou on it that holds Oliver's bookmarks. It became part of our Disney collection during our visit in 2013. Gaston's was the location of Oliver's 5th birthday breakfast: a cinnamon roll the size of Oliver's head with a LeFou's Brew. Joe and Oliver love sweets and this cinnamon roll has so much white creamy frosting they had to dig to find the actual roll. I'm more a savory girl, especially at breakfast, so I sat there feeling like a caveman gnawing on the meaty, also quite huge but nicely seasoned, pork shank, which sadly has been removed from the menu. It was replaced by more meat, but in the form of a tavern beef stew. Not quite as manly, but it comes with a hunk of baguette you can gnaw on.

Gaston's is perfectly themed. In the dining room you feel as if you have been transported into the movie, with oversized wooden chairs and tables and a large fireplace with a portrait of Gaston above the mantel. Outside the windows you can see the fountain where Belle enjoyed her books and a series of small buildings with cobblestone walkways. It's a picturesque corner of Fantasyland not to be missed.

Location Tip: Gaston's has two dining rooms and a few small tables outside as well. Try to sit in the dining room with the fireplace for a more authentic experience. It feels like you're in the scene in the movie, but tromping around wearing boots and biting in wrestling matches is frowned upon.

Grey Stuff

At Be Our Guest in the Magic Kingdom, the Grey Stuff is available for breakfast, lunch, and dinner. During breakfast and lunch, it's served atop the Master's Cupcake as a light, fluffy frosting with a hint of dark cocoa topped with little baubles of silver, copper, and gold that add crunch and contrast.

Ordering Tip: Make sure to read the dessert menu carefully to ensure you're ordering the dessert with the Grey Stuff. Some folks don't notice it as part of the description for the Master's Cupcake. At dinner the menu more clearly specifies the Grey Stuff as a separate item. If you're a picky eater, ask how the Grey Stuff will be served when ordering dinner.

For dinner, the pastry chef determines how the Grey Stuff will be served, and it can change from day to day. In May 2017, Nate and Sam had Mickey-shaped Grey Stuff topping a chocolate shell filled with a cookie crème (a custard-like creamy pudding). One Halloween, the Grey Stuff was sprinkled with tiny pumpkins, ghosts, and bats, and served atop a rich brownie.

The true highlight of any meal at Be Our Guest is the Grey Stuff. Sitting in a scene from the movie while eating a dish from the soundtrack is one of the most magical munching experiences at Disney World.

Grilled Cheese

Is grilled cheese one of your child's food groups? Disney understands and so grilled cheese is a staple on many restaurant menus at Disney World—with a little pixie dust, of course. In fact, over 80 restaurants feature some sort of grilled cheese, from the gourmet croque monsieur at Be Our Guest to the classic sandwich at the Plaza Restaurant in Magic Kingdom.

At The Wave at the Contemporary, grilled cheese comes on rainbow bread, which is a thick slice of white bread with a mix of colors not found in nature swirled into the bread dough. The colors are almost day-glo and look more like they should be in a set of Crayola markers, not something you should put in your stomach. Oliver loved it.

If you're looking for a healthy grilled cheese alternative, check out Whispering Canyon Café at Wilderness Lodge. Their grilled cheese is served on healthy multi-grain bread that gives it a satisfying crunch. The sandwich is cut into strips and comes with a side of tomato soup for dipping.

H

Harissa Chicken Roll

Harambe Market

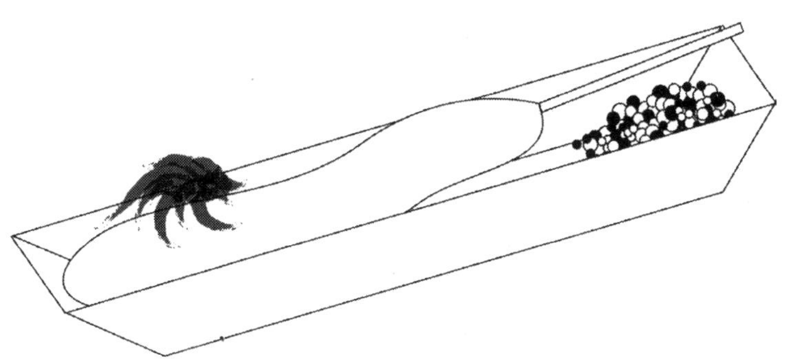

Harissa Chicken Roll

You can order a harissa chicken roll at Spice Road Table in the Morocco Pavilion at Epcot, and it has also made an appearance on the menu at Food & Wine Festival.

Best described as the Moroccan version of an egg roll, the outside is a crispy pastry with chicken, corn, cilantro, harissa and cheese on the inside. I love roasted red peppers, and this is a dominant flavor in Disney's harissa.

At Spice Road Table, the roll is served with a spicy ketchup that I thought added a bit too much of a kick and masked some of the fresher flavors from the red peppers.

Location Tip: Spice Road Table is a newer restaurant in the World Showcase and is located right on the lagoon. Its amazing view of the lagoon and of IllumiNations is still a bit of a hidden gem. If you want a seat, a cocktail, and some harissa with your fireworks, get a reservation for about an hour or so before IllumiNations starts.

Harambe Market

Harambe Market is an open-air quick-service location tucked into a corner of Animal Kingdom's Africa. It's open for lunch and dinner. The food is South African-inspired street food. There are four walk-up windows serving sausages, chicken, and even soda from Zimbabwe. There is ample seating. Head to the far back tables and get a glimpse of the train to Rafiki's Planet Watch as it chugs by.

Ordering Tip: If you need a grown-up way to cool off, head over to Dawa Bar and grab a cocktail before eating to Harambe.

One of the most popular dishes at Harambe is the beef and pork sausage. Think of a carnival corn dog, but instead of the county fair, it comes from Johannesburg. In appearance, it's a thin, (nearly) foot-long sausage fried in a curry batter. Everyone looks ridiculous eating it, but it's too tasty for anyone to care. The sausage is slightly spicy with a hint of sweetness from the curry batter. It's served with one or two small sides that change with the seasons. In the fall of 2015, it came with a broccoli salad. In the spring of 2017, it came with black-eyed pea salad and a carrot-jicama slaw. Most of the time the salad has a touch of vinegar, which balances out the sweetness from the curry batter. The black-eyed pea salad had tomatoes and little bursts of sweetness from the corn.

Ordering Tip: Every window at Harambe has the exact same menu. It's a bit deceiving because the menus on the wall may be different. Trust me, you can get the sausage at any of the four windows.

Tikka masala chicken, ribs, and chicken skewers are also on the menu. But the sausage is the dish. Even cast members love this treat: Nick says, "We get this every time we go to Animal Kingdom. It's huge! It's probably more than one person should eat, but it's a fun African take on an American classic."

Ordering Tip: The unusual soda flavors from Club Cool have found their way into Animal Kingdom. If the Dixie-size cup size offering at Club Cool of the raspberry cream sparberry from Zimbabwe wasn't enough, you can buy a vat (in the shape of a large, Disney-sized cup) of it here.

I

Ice Cream Bar, Mickey Shaped
Ice Cream Your Way
Inside a Disney Restaurant

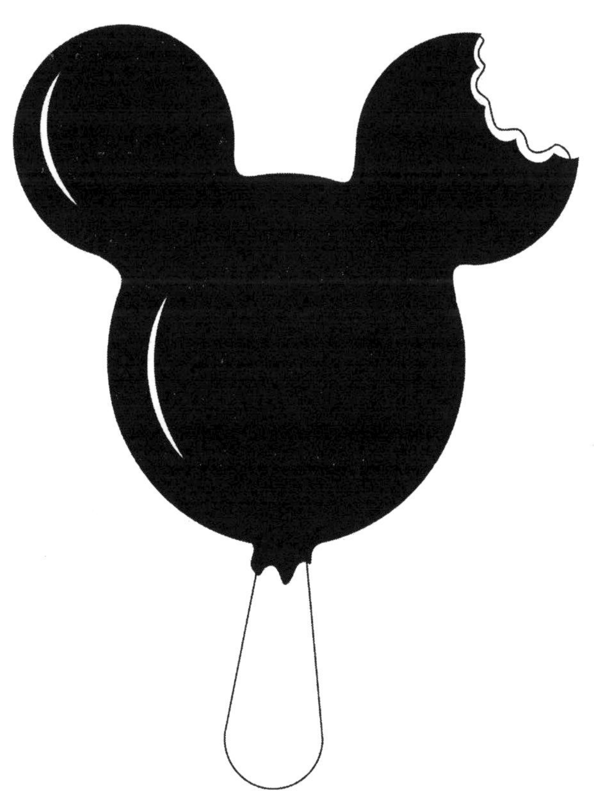

Ice Cream Bar, Mickey-shaped

Mickey ice cream bars are available year-round almost anywhere on Disney World property. It's also on Disney cruise ships, at every Disney park around the world, and if you're at a Disney resort that has a freezer in the store or in a quick-service restaurant, you might even be able to find one there. No other Disney treat has such widespread availability.

Ordering Tip: Mickey Ice cream bars are kept super cold. These things are frozen like a rock, but they need it to stand up to the Florida heat. If you have teeth sensitive to extreme cold, consider yourself warned.

Mickey ice cream bars are vanilla ice cream dipped in dark chocolate. The first bite is so delicious and crispy that it's no surprise that over 3.3 million of them are sold each year at Disney World alone.

Dining Tip: When it's Florida hot outside, eat them fast. It's a sad moment when a hunk of ice cream bar slides down your arm or globs onto your shoe.

If you were visiting Disney back in the 1980s, when these bars made their first appearance, they looked a bit different. Back then, instead of Mickey completely dipped in chocolate, the ears were chocolate ice cream and the rest was vanilla ice cream with a chocolate face in it.

What if sweets, ice cream, or dairy aren't your thing? No worries, you can still enjoy Mickey Ice cream bars. Here are just five of the many non-food ways to enjoy them:

- Magnets, for your fridge.
- Post-It notes, designed to resemble a Mickey ice cream bar with a little bite taken out of the ear.
- Shirts. Many different shirts feature this treat either alone or coupled with other Disney food favs like the turkey leg. My favorite is a shirt that is a pattern of small,

hand-drawn Disney World park icons: Cinderella Castle, Space Mountain, Tree of Life, Tower of Terror, turkey legs, and of course, Mickey ice cream bars. There is also a Disneyland version of the shirt.

- Chew toy. Now your favorite pet can have a safe way to munch on the iconic Disney treat.
- iPhone case.

Ice Cream Your Way

Kids love ice cream. Grown-ups, too. Getting to play pastry chef and choose your flavors and then pile up entirely too many sugary toppings is always a good time.

There are multiple places around Disney World where you can channel your inner dessert chef. In the Magic Kingdom, one of our family's favorites is the Ice Cream Bar at Crystal Palace a buffet-style restaurant that features character meals for breakfast, lunch, and dinner.

> **Location Tip**: At Crystal Palace, the ice cream bar is front and center. It might be a good idea to establish up front the amount of healthy food your kids need to eat before they can go nuts at the ice cream bar.

At The Wave in the Contemporary, they do things a little differently and in more reasonable portion sizes. Oliver loved the make-your-own sundae. He got to choose his ice cream flavor and they brought out a scoop in a glass bowl surrounded by smaller silver bowls with various toppings, the coolest being the bright, multi-colored Mickey sprinkles.

There are 14 different sundae options on the menu at Ghirardelli's in Disney Springs. If treats like Espresso Escape or Strike it Rich Butterscotch Hot Fudge Sundae lack appeal, and you want complete control of your ice cream, you can choose from over 10 flavors and 13 toppings to make your own.

One of the ultimate ice-cream adventures can be had at Beaches & Cream at Beach Club resort. There are many options on this menu including adult hard floats like the S'mores Float or the Stout Float featuring Guinness and chocolate sauce. But it's the Kitchen Sink at Beaches & Cream that puts this place on the ice-cream map. The Kitchen Sink has 6 types of ice cream and includes every topping they have. Every topping! This thing is just ginormous and has to be served in a small kitchen sink to fit the 10,000 or so calories of gluttony.

Inside a Disney Restaurant

If you've ever wondered what it's like behind the scenes at a Disney restaurant, here is your chance. Chef Lee worked at Liberty Tree Tavern in Magic Kingdom. From his training and funny reminders of working at Disney, to serving the best green beans every day, Chef Lee experienced a Disney kitchen first hand:

> Like every cast member you meet at Disney, chefs also go through the Disney Traditions training. The Disney training and experience changes your perspective on what Disney is about. In Traditions training, one of the first things they try to help you understand is that even though this is your job, for the guest, this may be a once-in-a-lifetime experience. Some families save up for years to spend four days at Disney. So every experience they have should be magical.
>
> During training, cast members at Liberty Tree learn that visiting the restaurant is a tradition in some families. There are grandparents that tell their grandkids that they went to Liberty Tree Tavern and they had the best Thanksgiving meal they ever had. When those grandchildren take their kids to Liberty Tree Tavern it must also be the best Thanksgiving dinner they have ever had. I took it to heart. Most cast members do. Disney really does try and get you to have that mindset, that all of the jobs, from the custodial staff, to characters and culinary staff, to entertainers, it's all on us to make it magical for the guest. So that first green bean I cooked had to be as good as the last one because every guest deserved the consistent, high-quality experience.

The challenge of being a chef at Disney is that in the average restaurant, you may serve 2500 people in a night. Cooking that volume in four hours time, to nail that dish every time in incredibly large quantities, is a huge challenge. For example, mashed potatoes. To make mashed potatoes for thousands of people, it required a giant floor mixer the size of one of the spinning teacups! The kitchen team would steam off trays and trays of potatoes then take them to a giant floor mixer, dump in giant pans of potatoes, gallons of milk, a salt mixture, and big pound blocks of butter. It was so fun. The sheer volume of making such large portions and still having it be good was a challenge, but the consistency had to be there. It's part of the magic of Disney.

There is so much camaraderie between all the cast members. Even though you're on show and on stage, these are all real people.

It was Disney's preference that cast members who aren't on stage aren't seen. Cast members enter the park in a non-public area. Some cast members go directly from the tunnels into the kitchen of a restaurant. Once in the kitchen, it feels just like most other restaurant kitchens. Then, there's the reminder. You're rushing to your shift and see Chip 'n' Dale bouncing down the hallway and then you're shocked, like, "Oh yeah, I work at Disney. There are two chipmunks over there." A kitchen is a kitchen and it's work, but it's when you're on break with a couple of princesses and a giant dog that you remember you're at Disney.

J

Jack Skellington Candy Apple

Jiko

Journals

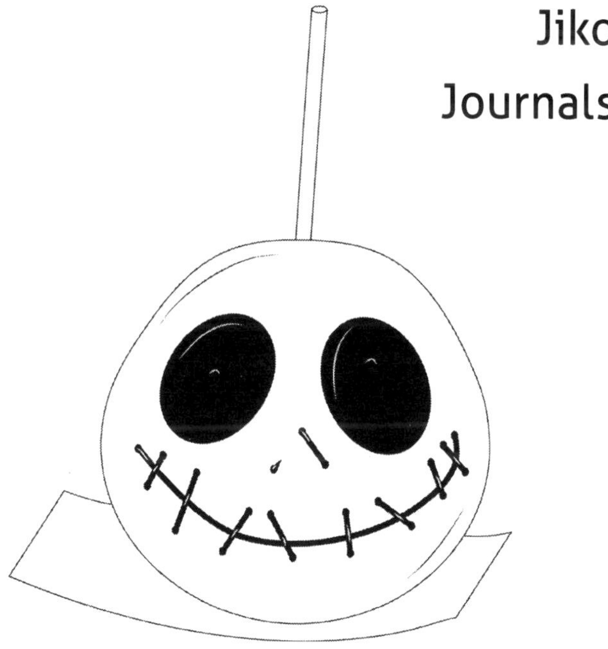

Jack Skellington Candy Apple

You can find Jack Skellington candy apples and similar seasonal treats at various locations around the parks and resorts. The best places to find holiday candy apples is at Main Street Confectionery and Big Top Treats at Magic Kingdom and Goofy's Candy Co at Disney Springs. There are treats for most major holidays from January to December, including Valentine's Day and St. Patrick's Day. But Disney pulls out all the stops for Halloween and Christmas.

During Halloween, the Poisoned Candy Apples are popular: bright red apples dipped in clear sugar syrup with green-white chocolate frosting covering the top of the apple, with ghoulish eyes, a nose, and a mouth. Eating one will make you feel just like Snow White with the Evil Queen hating your beauty.

A little less scary is the apple dipped in white chocolate that looks like a sweet Mickey ghost with a chocolate smiley face. There have also been Minnie witches with a purple witch hat, an orange bow, and Minnie's signature polka dot dress, with purple sprinkles and orange frosting spots. The man himself, Jack Skellington, is a white chocolate-dipped apple with Jack's face drawn on in midnight dark chocolate.

Location Tip: At the Magic Kingdom locations, you can watch the artisans at work decorating all the tasty treats. Main Street Confectionery has many treats, so it may be cake pops or cookies, not candy apples, on the decorating table. Big Top Treats in Fantasyland near the Dumbo ride has a nice viewing area and every time we have been there, candy apples were being decorated.

During Christmas, the standard Mickey and Minnie apples have Santa and Mrs. Claus hats. There are apples dipped in white chocolate drenched in blue, red, or green sprinkles with a white snowflake in white chocolate frosting. My favorite is the Mickey snowman with the apple dipped in white chocolate then dipped in white shiny sprinkles. The Mickey ears are two small marshmallows dipped in chocolate. The Mickey snowman is dressed for the season in festive scarf and chocolate candy eyes, nose, and buttons.

DISNEY FOOD CHALLENGE: Is it possible to try a new candy apple each month of the year? Check out the list below for a year of candy apples. Unless otherwise noted, visit Main Street Confectionery or Big Top Treats at Magic Kingdom or Goofy's Candy Co at Disney Springs for these apples.

- JANUARY: #Rock the Dots with the Minnie apple at Marceline's in Disney Springs.
- FEBRUARY: Share an apple with red hearts and white and dark chocolate frosting with someone you love.
- MARCH: Find the end of the rainbow with a Mickey ears leprechaun with a green sugar hat and pants.
- APRIL: Try the white chocolate bunny or bright yellow chicks in blue sprinkle eggs.
- MAY: Celebrate spring and WDW Gay Days with an apple coated in a rainbow of sprinkles.
- JUNE: Show Olaf what it's like at Disney in summer with the white chocolate Olaf candy apple.
- JULY: Be patriotic with a 4th of July apple coated in red, white, and blue sprinkles.
- AUGUST: The end of August marks the start of Halloween season at Disney. Channel your inner Snow White and start off with the Poisoned Apple.
- SEPTEMBER: Celebrate fall and Halloween with the bright orange Mickey Jack-o-Lantern candy apple.
- OCTOBER: Halloween is all about the costumes, so munch on Witch Minnie with her deep purple and orange polka-dot dress and witch's hat.
- NOVEMBER: Be thankful for Mickey and Minnie apples with red and green sprinkle outfits.
- DECEMBER: Do you want to eat a snowman? If it's a candy apple with chocolate Mickey ears and is covered in sparkly white sprinkles, yes!

Over 350 chefs work at Disney World, so it is possible that on your next trip one of these apples may not be available. No worries! There will be other ginormous apples smothered in sugary topping in their place.

Jiko

Jiko—The Cooking Place is an exotic signature-dining location at Animal Kingdom Lodge. It features the "tastes of Africa" and plating on par with fine dining experiences anywhere in the world. The elegant menu has dishes with African, Indian, and Mediterranean flavors. Jiko is only open for dinner, and if you are planning a dinner with a large group, Disney Dining will put you in contact directly with the restaurant.

Walking into Jiko is a play on the senses. The smell of meat and spices fills the air. The restaurant is decorated with dark wood furniture, deep red walls, and tiled columns. In the main dining room, there are white sculptures that seem as if they are in flight along the bright blue ceiling.

There is also a special room called the Wine Room. Being seated in this area doesn't always happen, so we felt lucky in 2015 when our party of 11 had this room almost to ourselves. The backdrop of our dinner was an ornate wall featuring an African pattern that looked as if it was carved of wood. The cast members are incredibly knowledgeable about the food and drink offerings. Our host was a lovely gentleman named Cornelius. He was from South Africa and had a beautiful accent. He was also very excited to practice speaking English (instead of his native Afrikaans) with all of our kids and visited us multiple times during the meal to talk about his favorite dishes.

In addition to interesting surroundings and authentic new foods, Jiko makes ordering your food a source of fun. Many of the dishes are quite exotic and it was amusing listening to Austin order lamb while trying to pronounce "ciabatta," Nickolas politely requesting a Nigerian-spiced pork chop, and Oliver asking, "May I have the steak with ancient grains, please?" There was also an extensive gluten-free menu for Maggie.

Make sure to try the African Table, a series of dips with kobz, poppy seed lavash, house-made naan. The Jiko salad is cool because it has greens from Epcot's Land Pavilion. There are a number of excellent South African wines to try, or you can be adventurous and order the sweet Zebratini. With rum, Godiva white chocolate liqueur, Frangelico, Amarula, and a shot of espresso in a zebra-striped martini glass, this is a wild (and dangerous) liquid dessert.

Our first trip to Jiko was after our Disney wedding in 2005. It had been so long ago and we were all so excited from the big day that we remembered little about the meal. To be able to go back in 2015 for our 10-year wedding anniversary with our bigger family was a magical treat.

There were a number of delicious-sounding appetizers, and we made the difficult decision of having the African Table and Indugay Tibs in Brik. If the Indugay Tibs In Brik sounds like a group of random syllables strung together, it was that way for us, too. It's a deep-fried pastry with seasonal fillings.

Dinner was a lot of pork love, with five people ordering the pork shank with apple butter. Annie and I decided to do African tapas and shared the boar tenderloin, maize soup, and the lobster tail with Madagascar vanilla bean poached butter. The lobster was perfectly cooked and the vanilla brought out the sweetness in the lobster meat. My favorite was the sweet maize soup with a dollop of red peppery creaminess from a harissa crème fraîche, meaty blue crab, and a burst of sweetness and freshness from roasted corn. We fought over the crunchy Dhania biscuit that when eaten with a spoonful of soup had a crunch that was a delight for the taste buds.

Ordering Tip: Ask your server for recommendations. Jiko's menu changes regularly to feature the freshest seasonal ingredients.

The dessert menu featured even more new vocabulary words. The catchy sounding malva pudding is a very fancy crème with cherries, crunchy toasted meringue, and a brandied cherry ice cream that added a brightness to balance the tartness from the cherries. Another favorite was the pot de crème, which is kind of like a crème brulee without the crunchy top. Annie went with the Valrhona chocolate mousse with a hazelnut dacquoise cake with strawberries and basil. This was renamed the Nutella dessert as it was passed around the table. I'm a salty-with-my-sweet girl and went with the cheese plate. It paired quite nicely with the sweet strawberries from Annie and crunchy lemony meringue from the malva pudding.

One of the chefs at Jiko is now head chef at Tiffins in Animal Kingdom. The menus are different, but the chef brought the tongue twister chakalaka with him to Tiffins, which is as fun to say as it is to eat.

Journals

In addition to those autographs books and PhotoPass photos, keeping a food journal is a fun and delicious way to remember your Disney trip. There are many different kinds of journals for kids of all ages to document all the tasty munchies adding magic to your Disney World vacation.

In our kids' journals, we have found Oliver's first taste of a cookie from Main Street Confectionery at Magic Kingdom, Austin experiencing the belly dancer while munching on beef brewat rolls at Restaurant Marrakesh in Epcot, and Maggie missing gluten during our trip to the Food & Wine Festival.

Our senses of smell and taste are a huge part of triggering memories, so try a food journal to accompany all those Instagram and Facebook posts.

K

Kiddie Cocktails

Kona Café

Kungaloosh Beer

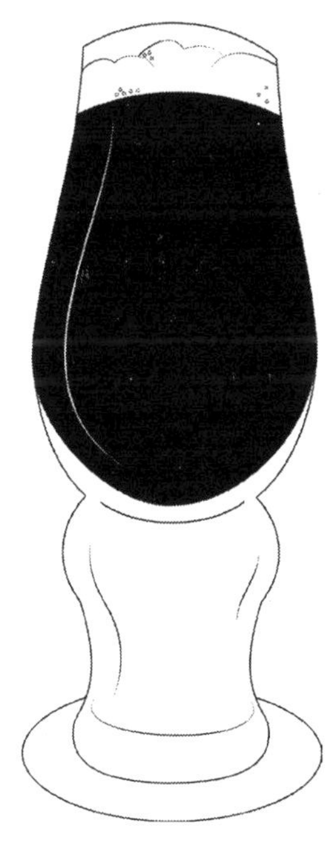

Kiddie Cocktails

"Kiddie cocktails" are available at any well-stocked Disney bar. The typical cocktail consists of Sprite with a shot of Grenadine. It's a non-alcoholic mixer that tastes a bit like red Kool-Aid. They're often served with a cherry or three.

This is Austin's signature drink. At most meals we always do a quick toast and having one of these in hand helps our kids feel like part of the toasting festivities.

Ordering Tip: Most of the time the kiddie cocktail is served with the traditional bright red maraschino cherry. Actual maraschino cherries are a much darker red, almost brown. They have a more natural and real cherry flavor.

In 2015, during our lunch at Sanaa, Annie ordered a kiddie cocktail and Nickolas ordered a Shirley Temple. Then it was Austin's turn. All the names had been used, so the Cast Member offered the "more grown-up alternative. Just order a Sprite with Grenadine. It sounds much more like an actual cocktail name," she suggested.

Now at every family meal when multiple kids go to order a kiddie cocktail, it's ordered three ways. We all smile and remember our magical meal at Sanaa. Then we all start talking about how we miss the Sanaa naan bread. And the giraffes. And then Disney in general.

Kona Café

Kona Café is in the Great Ceremonial House, the main building at the Polynesian Resort. It's open for breakfast, lunch, and dinner with a menu full of American favorites with a touch of Asian flavor.

The best way to get to Kona Café is to take the monorail, which will deposit you at the entrance to the resort. Taking a monorail to a resort is always cool because one minute you're zooming along outside and the next you're transported to a new world in a beautifully themed resort.

The Polynesian is tropical, huge, and smells like vacation. It has a great gift shop and is busy—too busy for my taste. The restaurant has bright lighting and high ceilings, and it's smack dab in the middle of a high traffic area, so it is very loud.

Location Tip: Have a dinner reservation for Kona around 7:30 or 8pm and then head down to the beach to watch the nighttime show at Magic Kingdom. The beach offers a great view for the fireworks, but the projections are a bit harder to see. The music and narration are piped through speakers on the beach. This is also one of the best spots to see the Electrical Water Pageant Parade.

During 2015 we ate our last meal of our trip at Kona Café. After the intimacy and upscale experiences of Jiko and Be Our Guest, it was a bit jolting. Our table was in the middle of the dining room, along the main walkway to the kitchen and to enter and exit the restaurant. It was the opposite of an intimate family dinner.

If the sea calls you like it does Moana, definitely head to Kona Café. Seafood is a specialty and many guests consider it the best place on Disney World property for sushi. Like any good sushi restaurant, the plating is beautiful and includes decorative elements. Our sushi plates featured bright purple flowers and intricately arranged vegetables.

By this point in the trip, everyone was tired and ready for a taste of something familiar. Quite a few folks ordered sushi, Joe had a Kona coffee-rubbed pork, and Oliver went with a taste of home, a hot dog.

Make sure to try the Kona crab cakes and a beer from Hawaii-based Kona Brewing Company. This is also the place where you can get a little taste of Moana with Te Fiti's Island Mousse.

The Polynesian is worth a visit and watching the fireworks glitter across the water at the beach is a great place to find the magic.

Kungaloosh Beer

This specialty beer is served year-round in the Animal Kingdom at Nomad's Lounge and Tiffins, in Africa, and (usually) at the Thirsty River Bar & Trek Snacks, in Asia.

Kungaloosh Beer, or Kungaloosh Spiced Excursion Ale Draft, is the first beer brewed exclusively for Disney World. It's a deep amber ale inspired by the adventures of Joe Rohde and the team of Imagineers that are behind all the magic at Animal Kingdom. Cardamom and cinnamon are just two of the spices included in the special blend.

My husband Joe is our beer drinker and described Kungaloosh as hoppy with a clean finish and depth of flavor. He loves cardamom so much we regularly have cardamom and sugar for topping toast at home. He was looking for a bit more cardamom, but said it's good enough to order again. If there's a beer drinker in your group, make sure to quaff a Kungaloosh.

L

Large Krispy Head

Les Chefs de France

Liberty Tree Tavern

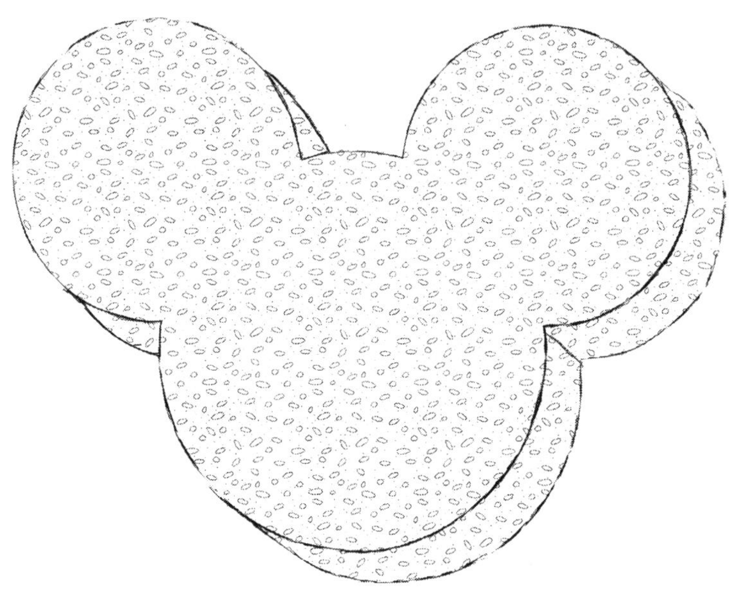

Large Krispy Head

This colossal Rice Krispy treat in the shape of Mickey's head can be found at Main Street Confectionery in Magic Kingdom. It is so massive that it costs around $15–20 and the nutritional label doesn't give an official weight. It definitely weighs at least a pound. That may not sound like a lot, but eight wrapped Rice Krispy treats you find at the grocery store come in at less than a pound. Eight of them are less than just one large krispy head. Trust me, it's a whole lot of krispy.

Normal-size krispy treats are one of those Disney staples that get the character and seasonal treatment, like candy apples. These smaller treats typically come on a stick. They're the mini-me versions of the large krispy head, for which no stick is big enough—maybe a branch.

At Goofy's Candy Company in Disney Springs, the normal-sized krispy treats are lathered in candies, drizzled in chocolate, and even dipped in M&Ms. During the holidays, there is an adorable Santa version with red sprinkles, a fluffy white marshmallow, and white chocolate frosting for Santa's suit.

The craziest krispy treat is one that masquerades as another iconic Disney food: the turkey leg. Seriously. It's in the shape of a turkey leg with milk chocolate frosting and a touch of white chocolate frosting at the end to represent the bone. And of course it's gluten-free and vegetarian, too.

Here's a great way to mess with your head. Buy the Turkey Leg Krispy and then go stand next to one of the turkey leg stands so you get all the juicy meat smells. Then take the first bite of your treat. It's a fun reminder of how your brain connects sight and smell with taste. Whether it's Santa, turkey legs, or a Mickey's head that is larger than your own, krispy treats are some major magical munching.

Les Chefs de France

Les Chefs de France, serving French bistro food, is located at the main thoroughfare or promenade of Epcot's France Pavilion.

Chef Bruno, its head chef, says, "Our food is authentic French food. The only difference is that the portion size is larger." Les Chefs has been at Epcot since the park opened in October 1982. Chef Bruno, who was born in France and is a classically trained chef, has been there since then, providing Epcot guests with a traditional French dining experience.

Like many restaurants sprinkled throughout the France Pavilion, Les Chefs serves one of the most traditional French bistro dishes, steak frites, a flat iron steak in a lemon and butter sauce with thin crispy French fries. Now, in France the steak would be rare or even medium rare, but as Chef Bruno says, "People come here and ask for and expect French food, but we have to make and cook dishes people here will like." So that means if you want your steak frites well done, Chef Bruno and his team will accommodate you.

In addition to the scrumptious lobster bisque and the delicious variety of gourmet offerings in the assiette campagnarde (charcuterie), there are multiple seafood options. The traditional salade niçoise is filled with ahi tuna, tomato, green beans, and hard-boiled eggs. "The salad of my city," shared Mallorie, a cast member from Nice, France, who works here, "except at home we would use canned tuna, which is not as good as the tuna here!"

If you're like the 3,000 or so other guests each day that have the crossiant escargots at Food & Wine and want a fix between festivals, try the cassoulette escargots.

One of our family's favorite dishes is the flatbreads. The tomat et fromage de chevre has a European-style super-thin cracker-like crust topped with tangy tomato sauce, fresh basil, and earthy goat cheese. Some guests swear by the pizza at Via Napoli in the Italy Pavilion, but the flatbreads at Les Chefs are bang on for thin-crust fans. I know how much everyone loved this flatbread because we have photographic evidence of 8-year old Annie looking longingly at Nate biting into his flatbread during our 2005 trip.

Ordering Tip: Ask your server for suggestions. All of the servers are from France and experts on the food. Many have favorite dishes on the menu that are famous in their city or village. You may be able to try a dish from the server's childhood like gratin de macaroni. Or be entertained by a story about how soupe à l'oignon gratinée is the hangover food of France. No White Castle or Taco Bell for the French, it's an onion at the back of the fridge and some day-old crusty baguette!

There are three different dining areas. A sunroom at the back that overlooks the fountain and the Beauty and the Beast topiaries on display during the Flower & Garden festival. A sunroom at the front overlooks the promenade along the Seven Seas Lagoon and has what Chef Bruno calls "one of the best restaurant views in Epcot." The middle dining room has booths and tables and gives a more traditional French bistro feel. On almost every trip to Epcot we visit Les Chefs and have had the pleasure of dining in all three rooms.

Location Tip: For most months of the year, Serveur Amusant performs just outside the windows at the front of the restaurant. If you sit in the front sunroom, you will have a full view of the amazing acrobatics. The performer will stack chairs 3–4 high on a table and perform handstands and feats of strength. It's dinner and a show all in one.

The cast members are the best part of this restaurant. Everyone is from France and has a ton of passion for their homeland and its food. We have met so many lovely CM's at Les Chefs, including Lido, a waiter who speaks six different languages; Mallorie, who shared all of her favorite dishes and stories of her time managing Le Halles Boulangerie; and Chef Bruno, who remembers a Disney World before Animal Kingdom and an Epcot when there was no Test Track or Mission: SPACE. We have been eaten at nearly four dozen different locations around Disney World, but the team of hard-working and passionate cast members at Les Chefs delivers a dining experience that is one of the best and most magical we've found.

Liberty Tree Tavern

Liberty Tree Tavern, in Liberty Square at the Magic Kingdom, serves American comfort foods. Dinner is Thanksgiving with a traditional family-style turkey dinner with all the trimmings. You can choose from different dining rooms that are historically themed for different American heroes, including George Washington, Betsy Ross, and Benjamin Franklin. In 2016 the restaurant added grown-up beverages to the menu, putting the "tavern" into Liberty Tree Tavern.

Chef Lee, a former chef at Liberty Tree Tavern, says:

> The lunch menu was great. It was much more varied and there are a lot more options than the dinner menu. At lunch you can get delicious sandwiches, crunchy salads, or comforting pot roast.
>
> Dining here is really about the experience. It's colonial, set in a specific time period, and the theming reflects that. The meal is about enjoying a big family-style meal, being very laid back, and having fun with your server. The restaurant is fairly loud and there were always lots of kids. Family-style restaurants at Disney tend to be loud.
>
> Our sides at Liberty Tree Tavern were super good. The green bean recipe is one I still make at home today. It's so simple, just the beans, butter, salt, and pepper. The menu also featured a spring squash-vegetable medley with a seasoning of celery salt, pepper, and garlic salt. The mix of zucchini, yellow squash, and red onion with that seasoning mix was so good. It was fun and a challenge cooking it in a large volume to get it just right, tender enough but with a little bit of snap to it. Mushy, overcooked zucchini and squash are not okay.

Liberty Tree Tavern is one of the best restaurants if you're at Disney for Thanksgiving or Christmas. Or if you're a history enthusiast. Or it's May and you're craving a traditional Thanksgiving meal of turkey with all the fixings. Or if you're a Hamilton fan and want to run into the George Washington room and start singing "Here Comes the General."

M

Marketplaces at Epcot International Food & Wine Festival

Mickey-shaped Foods

Mugs

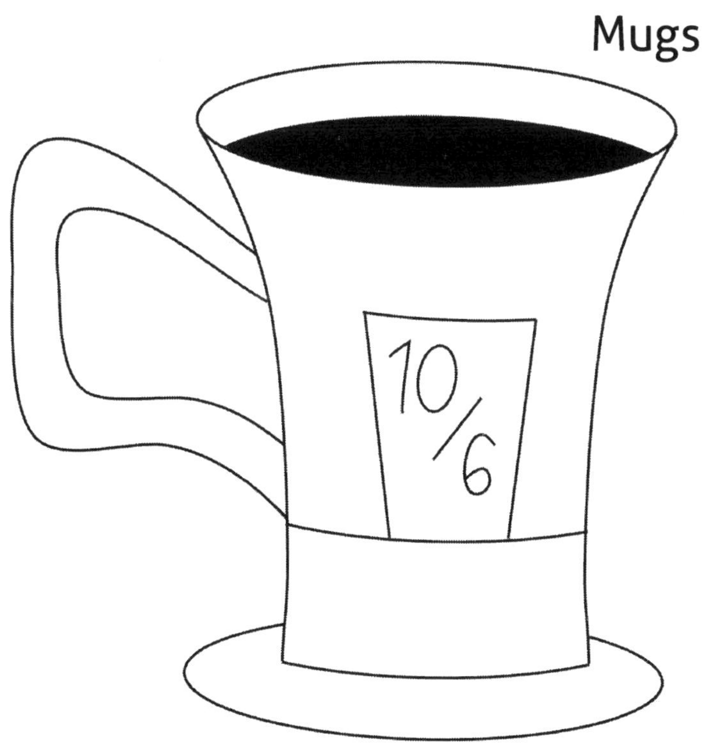

Marketplaces at Epcot International Food & Wine Festival

Marketplaces are the name of the food kiosks at the Epcot International Food & Wine Festival, the event which started the food festival craze at Epcot. Once Disney saw how much guests loved visiting the different food kiosks for tastes from all over the world, they added the food kiosks to Flower & Garden and to the International Festival of the Holidays. Food & Wine is all about trying new tastes from the approximately 95 different dishes available.

There were 35 different marketplaces in 2017 to celebrate Epcot's 35th anniversary. Each marketplace offered 2-3 dishes, wines, beers, and often at least one signature cocktail like the Snow Shadow at the Japan Marketplace. Food & Wine is akin to visiting gourmet restaurants in cities around the world—cities that you can walk through, with a drink in your hand.

On a non-festival day at Epcot you can sample cuisines from 11 different countries just by visiting the World Showcase pavilions. During Food & Wine the number of countries is over 20 and includes exotic locations like Patagonia and Thailand. One of the things many guests rave about is the selection of different dishes and the unique cocktails at the festival.

Food & Wine ran for a record 75 days in 2017. The festival is constantly changing and the marketplaces and the food and drink offerings at each marketplace also change each year. In 2016 there were five new marketplaces, with a few from the previous year, including the Dominican Republic, that didn't come back. In 2017 it was all about bringing back old favorites.

What marketplace on a busy day sold almost 3,000 of one of their food items? The France Marketplace has been home to the crossaint aux escargot for a few years. According to Chef Bruno, the head chef of Les Chefs de France, it is the most popular and best-selling dish at the entire Food & Wine Festival. Chef Bruno would know, as all the prep work for the dish is completed in his kitchen, with assembly and final plating done at the marketplace.

It is the chefs at the restaurants in each country in the World Showcase who determine what dishes will be on offer at the Marketplaces. This means that sometimes you will see World Showcase restaurant favorites at a marketplace. This happened in Morocco in 2016 when the famous hummus fries from Spice Road Table were at the Morocco Marketplace.

Thirty-five marketplaces, four coffee carts, and a few other festival locations were spread throughout Epcot in 2017. At the other three festivals, Disney has a bit more fun with the food kiosk names. At Food & Wine, however, the marketplace names are more straightforward, usually just the country. Here are all the marketplaces from 2017 with a few dishes and cocktails that stood out—and may be back for 2018:

- Active Eats was new in 2017 and was the place to fuel up to make it through the rest of the festival. There was a roasted salmon with quinoa salad and a loaded mac and cheese with bacon. All good things include bacon. One of my favorite tastes from Festival of the Holidays made its Food and Wine appearance in dessert form: the avocado crema with strawberries, yellow cake, and tortilla streusel. The drink offerings were a few different festival wines and just when you thought they couldn't do anything else to water, this Marketplace had hard sparkling water.
- Africa was back with dishes like gluten-free Berbere-style beef tenderloin with jalapenos and pap, and a spicy Ethiopian red lentil stew with yogurt. Were you brave enough to try the stew the traditional Ethiopian way, and eat it with your hands? Maybe after a few African wines.
- Almond Orchard was new in 2017 and was all about those heart-healthy nuts, almonds. With a banana almond sundae with berries and dark chocolate, it may be sort of heart-healthy, but not so diet-friendly. If bubbles were your thing, Almond Orchard satisfied your needs with three different champagnes.
- Australia maintained its status as one of the best marketplaces to find gluten-free dishes. In 2015, Maggie really enjoyed the gluten-free grilled sweet-and-spicy bushberry shrimp with pineapple, pepper, onion, and snap peas.

The shrimp was perfectly grilled, the toppings offered an interesting mix of flavors, and the sauce added a nice zing. The grilled lamb chop with mint pesto and potato crunchies is also gluten-free. Sadly, the lamington cake was not gluten-free, but this yellow cake dipped in chocolate and shredded coconut is vegetarian and yummy. Many guests who made the trek over to the Chocolate Studio for a gluten-free dessert first grabbed a glass of Australian shiraz or ale here.

- Belgium is a country without a World Showcase pavilion. Its marketplace served two beers: a Hoegaarden and a Leffe blonde. Not surprisingly, a Belgian waffle was on the menu, served with either chocolate ganache or berry compote. Belgium also served a beer-braised beef with smoked gouda mashed potatoes.
- Block & Hans was one of the two marketplaces in the American Adventure Pavilion. Beer and cider dominated the menu. Those not into beer or cider could try Frozen Spiked Tea with Orange Vodka.
- Brazil is another country not in the World Showcase, so it's a special treat to have Brazilian dishes during Food & Wine. In 2015, we sampled the escondidinho de carne ("Little Hidden One"), layered meat pie with mashed yucca. It was kind of boring. Brazilian food is typically delicious, but this meat pie was in a bowl with decently flavored ground beef, similar to a homemade taco, and a sad dollop of hardened mashed potatoes. On the flip side, the frozen caipirinha was very refreshing cocktail that featured cachaça, the famous Brazilian pure sugar cane spirit that makes mixed drinks quite dangerous. Were it not for the $10 price tag and the small portion size, I would have set up shop at the Brazil Marketplace. Both of these items were still on the menu in 2017.
- Brewer's Collection, near the Germany Pavilion, was home to German beers, including a beer flight. For the romantics in your group, there was lebkuchenherz, a decorated gingerbread heart.

- Canada once again served the Canadian cheese soup, a festival favorite. With one of the most popular Epcot restaurants being Le Cellier, Canada typically has a meat dish. The "Le Cellier" wild mushroom beef filet with truffle butter could be enjoyed with a lager or apple ice wine.
- The Cheese Studio was back. Cheese in pasta. Cheese in a tart. And of course, a cheese trio. On the must-try list was the strawberry macaron with boursin pepper cheese. Few things go better with cheese than wine!
- China was once again home to the Beijing roast duck steamed bun. This bite was like a Chinese taco. On the outside it's a chewy white bun, similar to fancy Wonder Bread, and inside is duck with a crispy skin. Hoisin sauce adds a bit of sweet and spicy to the dish. China also had black pepper shrimp with Sichuan noodles and a spicy chicken dish. You could combat all that spice with a number of cocktails like the BaiJoe Punch with bai jui spirit and coconut, or the Ritzy Lychee with vodka and Courvoisier.
- The Chocolate Studio was new in 2016 and was back in 2017. There seemed to be some Festival of the Arts food influence here with a side called Raspberry Dust. In addition to that, the marketplace offered Liquid Nitro Chocolate with almond truffle and warm whiskey caramel and a sweet dark chocolate raspberry torte. Both paired well with Rosa Regale, a sparkling red wine.
- Coastal Eats was new in 2017 and had more than a few ways to enjoy some fruits of the sea. Crab cake with avocado lemongrass cream and baked shrimp scampi made crustacean-loving guests happy. The happiest guests paired their seafood with Pinots from Oregon.
- Craft Beers stepped up their food game with a chilled Scotch egg with sausage and mustard sauce. Few things go better with beer than burgers, so there was also a zesty cheeseburger and macaroni handwich. Even cotton candy went upscale with a l'orange cotton candy. This was a must-hit marketplace for beer lovers with the Florida Beer Company's chocolate milk stout.

- Earth Eats was this year's marketplace inspired by *The Chew* television series. In previous years it was Chew Lab and Chew Collective. It once again merged fresh flavors and technology with a ricotta and zucchini ravioli and a peanut butter and white chocolate mousse with caramel drizzle. They also had "celebrity wines" from Kurt Russell's vineyard.
- Farm Fresh borrowed some of the flavor profiles from the Flower & Garden Festival Outdoor Kitchens with a roasted beet salad with feta cheese and walnuts. There were also a variety of hard ciders with flavors like raspberry and elderberry cream, as well as a hard cider flight.
- Flavors from Fire was the place for those who complain that "it's not spicy enough!" The Piggy Wings with Korean BBQ sauce from Craft Beers took up residence here, alongside a sweet pancake with spicy chipotle chicken sausage. This marketplace even brought the heat to dessert with its chocolate picante: dark chocolate mousse with cayenne pepper, chili pepper, raspberry dust. There was liquid spice with the Smokin' Blackwater Porter and the Peppery Zinfandel.
- France is known for its very popular croissant aux escargots, but their marketplace also typically features a crème brulee. Its flavor tends to change each year and for 2017 it was la confiture de framboises: crème brulee with house-made raspberry jam. France offered a few different wines, but the most popular cocktail is the Ice Pop, a frozen boozy popsicle. In 2016, the Ice Pop flavor was strawberry with Caribbean Rhum Clement, but 2017 it was back to La Passion Martini Slush with Le Citron, cranberry, and passion fruit juice.
- Germany had a tongue-twister dish called schinkennudeln: a pasta gratin with ham and cheese. Bratwurst on a pretzel roll was also on the menu along with apple strudel. The marketplace featured a few different wines, including some varietals of Riesling.
- Greece made a play on an American classic, but took it vegan with its loaded Greek nachos with meatless sausage

and vegan tzatziki sauce. New this year was the Taste of Greece platter with stuffed grape leaves, grilled octopus, and feta cheese dip. A number of Greek wines were available that transported drinkers to the beautiful blue waters and rooftops of Santorini.

- Hawaii was all about the pineapple with a kalua pork slider with sweet-and-sour Dole pineapple chutney and a sparkling pineapple wine to pair it with. Festival-goers looking for the most famous pineapple-flavored item at Disney World, Dole Whip, headed over to the Refreshment Port.
- Hops & Barley at American Adventure brought back its venerable New England lobster roll, and also offered beef brisket with pimento cheese on garlic toast with a Cold-Brew Coffee Pilsner or a Cuvee red blend to wash it down.
- India was back! Food & Wine fans celebrated with pistachio cardamom bundt cake and two dishes incorporating naan: korma chicken with cucumber tomato salad and warm naan with pickled garlic and mango salsa. Namaste!
- Ireland's food stuck to the ribs, especially the roasted Irish sausage with colcannon potatoes and onion gravy. The warm chocolate pudding with Irish cream liqueur custard returned. Ireland had multiple drink offerings, including a frozen Twinings pumpkin chai tea with vodka–also available in a shake version for those under 21.
- Islands of the Caribbean featured four tropical-inspired dishes, including a gluten-free mojo pork with black beans, cilantro rice and pickled red onions, and a vegetarian quesito puff pastry with sweetened cream cheese and guava sauce. Cocktail fans imbibed the island flavors with a frozen mojito or Caribbean sangria.
- Italy had the one of the most extensive wine selections of the marketplaces. The chefs ensured that there will be a few wines that paired nicely with dishes like crispy calamari or costoletta di agnello alla marchigiana (braised T-bone lamb chops with onions, thyme, and lamb jus). Italy went all new in 2017 on every dish except its classic cannoli with sweet ricotta and candied fruit.

- Japan featured a few new dishes: the salmon BLT roll and wasabi shumai steamed pork dumplings. Fingers crossed that some day the adorable Tokyo Disney shumai that look like the little aliens from *Toy Story* make an appearance. Japan offered a few sakes to try and this year there were two sake cocktails: Pom Pineapple and Snow Shadow.
- Light Lab kept guests refreshed all day with its science-inspired cocktails. Kids came here for the mocktails: T=CC2 (vanilla tonic water with cotton candy) and the RGB citrus apple Freeze. There was also Boba Pearls in Cuvee and Space Dust Beer. Live long and prosper.
- Mexico had our second favorite taste in 2015, the tacos de camaron. In 2017, the taco dish was rib eye on a corn tortilla. Festival foodies indulged their sweet tooth with the new cajeta mousse with cajeta sauce and white chocolate flakes. Each year Mexico has a special margarita on the rocks flavor: 2015 was guava, 2016 featured both jalapeno and pineapple, and 2017 was prickly pear and a classic pomegranate.
- Morocco is my favorite pavilion in World Showcase and their restaurants offer dishes with exotic flavors that are challenging and new. In 2016, the Morocco Marketplace offered spicy hummus fries, a popular item offered at Spice Road Table, and it was back in 2017. This year's dessert was a chocolate baklava. With its fairly central location in World Showcase, Morocco was a popular stop to grab a refreshing cocktail like Moroccan sangria or Casa beer.
- New Zealand was not quite as special-diet-friendly as its Australian neighbor, but its lamb meatball with spicy tomato chutney and steamed green lip mussels with toasted breadcrumbs was equally tasty. New in 2017 was a frozen wine cocktail.
- Patagonia is a place most guests have not visited and is a popular marketplace stop. The menu included a beef empanada and a gluten-free grilled beef skewer with chimichurri sauce and boniato puree. Red wine fans smiled big purple smiles with Pinot noir and Malbec wines.

- Refreshment Cool Outpost, near the Africa Marketplace, offered a spicy hot dog with kimchi slaw and mustard sauce. The Cape Mountain and the Whiskey Frozen Coke were the perfect relaxing pick me ups to get festival-goers to their next port of call.
- Refreshment Port, near Showcase Plaza, was Dole Whip HQ at Epcot. The traditional Dole Whip was available, as well as a grown-up version with Bacardi coconut rum. It was like vacation in a cup. Refreshment Port also had a croissant doughnut with cinnamon and sugar, and fried chicken chunks with Dole pineapple sweet-and-sour sauce. But really, most guests went there for the boozy Dole Whip.
- Scotland is home to dishes with the words neeps, tatties, and the Tipsy Laird, a whiskey-soaked cake with lemon cream and toasted oats. It shared the menu with the Citrus Thistle with Hendricks Gin. Scotland was a good place to be if you're gluten-free with its fresh potato pancake with Scottish smoked salmon. And of course, there was Scotch, separately and as part of a flight.
- Spain made its way back into Food & Wine, tapas style, with Charcuterie in a Cone, a selection of Spanish meats, cheese, and olives. The paella was gluten-free and bursting with shrimp, mussels, and crispy chorizo. For dessert: sweet olive oil cake with powdered sugar and lemon curd, along with various Spanish wines.
- Thailand had been gone for 8 years, but was back in 2017 and ready to amaze mouths with red hot spicy Thai curry beef. There was also a seared shrimp with scallop cake and a cold noodle salad. A German Gewürztraminer wine and Singha lager helped cool down from the bold flavors.
- Showcase Coffee Carts were dotted throughout the festival. Each of the four carts offered their own grown-up cocktail. The coffee cart between the UK and Canada served a Kahula-tini and the one near American Adventure had a taste of summer with a Strawberry-Lemon Sunset.
- Wine & Dine Studio was competing with Italy for the number of wine offerings. To soak up some of their wines,

there was pulled duck confit with cannellini bean ragout with a Zinfandel reduction or a trio of artisan cheeses. There was also the fun plating of the Artist Palette of Wine and Cheese. This dish resembled a painter's palette with small holes for the wine and the cheeses were artistically spread across the palette.

In another lesson in how the magic is always changing, one of our favorite kiosks from 2015 and 2016, South Korea, was missing in 2017. Just have to make those delicious roasted pork lettuce wraps at home.

If all the walking isn't your speed and there is room in your vacation budget for next time, try the Party for the Senses. At this popular shindig, you can try dishes from the chefs at countless Disney restaurants at parks from around the world as well as dishes from some of the best chefs from around the country. This event is all you can eat and drink, and for the right price you even get reserved seating. No more balancing your plate of gourmet food on your knees.

Every year at Food & Wine there are also many special events in restaurants in Epcot and at restaurants around Disney World, so you could probably stay the entire festival and not eat the same thing twice ... unless it's the croissant aux escargot from France or the spicy hummus fries from Morocco.

Mickey-shaped Foods

Mickey-shaped foods dominate breakfast, lunch, dinner, and snacks at Disney World. You can find them just about anywhere in the parks, at the resorts, and even in various non-food formats.

In addition to ice cream, pretzels, and waffles, there are cookies in Mickey shapes, especially gingerbread men with Mickey ears during holiday time. Ice cream sundaes are made more special with brightly colored Mickey sprinkles at places like The Wave at the Contemporary Resort. Mickey ears appear on cupcakes at Main Street Confectionery and the Fireworks Dessert Party at Magic Kingdom. Sweet Mickey-shaped treats prevail with lollipops and candy and many treats are found at Goofy's Candy Company at Disney Springs.

Mickey-shaped food is a trendsetter and Disney continues to offer more and more ways to eat your favorite characters. During Star Wars weekends, Hollywood Studios has had Chips and Sith, where you can attack the Sith head dip with your Jedi chips. For the launch of *Guardians of the Galaxy 2*, guests took a bite out of Baby Groot's adorable head in bread form at Disneyland. Even Olaf became a tasty treat during Frozen fever at Disney World. As bizarre as this whole practice may be, these treats get major airtime on social media and the more cute and popular the character, the more people love to eat it.

Mugs

Mugs are available at most Disney restaurants and stores, and in many varieties. Some come with free refills, some light up, and at Disney Springs you can get them with boozy drinks, and others are just really cute.

Refillable mugs can be purchased at most Disney resorts and are good for free refills at any Disney resort. They traditionally have a Disney World design. When you purchase this mug, you get free refills of soda, coffee, teas, and hot chocolate.

Disney Springs has a mug/souvenir cup program. Each of the major restaurants in Disney Springs has a cup for grown-ups and a different one for kids. This way a grown-up can walk around with a tipple from their favorite Disney Springs restaurant. Each of the participating Disney Springs locations has a different design for their cup or mug and some restaurants go all out, like a lighthouse design for BOATHOUSE, a Splitsville bowling pin, or the understated gingham design for Chef Art Smith's Homecomin'.

Each park has different souvenir mugs and cups on offer. There are no free refills, but they are a fun souvenir item that has the benefit of containing a refreshing beverage. Sometimes called Souvenir Sippers, these items are constantly changing, so if you see one you can't live without, buy it, or else risk paying a premium later on eBay. The cups are themed for the seasons.

When a new movie is released, you can bet you will be drinking from a vessel designed to promote the movie. Hollywood

Studios is home to Star Wars and superheroes, and the cutest mug/cup award goes to the Baby Groot cup. The top is little Groot with moveable arms and the cup is his flowerpot. The Chewbecca beer stein at the Star Wars Dessert Party is designed so you open Chewy's head to take a drink. Magic Kingdom has different mugs/cups in each land, including a LeFou's Brew stein at Gaston's Tavern and two of the most popular mugs: the Country Bear Jamboree jug and the Orange Bird sipper.

Epcot has souvenir mugs for each of the festivals. Flower & Garden 2017 was a coffee mug that looked like a flowerpot. It wasn't in-the-park-practical, but great for the gardener in your life. The most popular Epcot mug is the beer stein found in a number of the pavilions, including Canada and Germany. Animal Kingdom doesn't have as many souvenir mugs as the other parks, but when they do, they do it right, such as a collapsible paper lantern and a color-changing mug that resembled an ornate oil lamp.

Don't forget the resorts! A few resort restaurants and lounges have some of the most coveted and well-known mugs, in particular the ones available at Trader Sam's Grog Grotto in the Polynesian. The Shrunken Zombie and the Polynesian Pearl are served in super-cool souvenir mugs that will take up a decent amount of room in your suitcase. And if you've run out of room, you can shop for mugs from the comfort of your home on disneystore.com.

So, if you're going to be ordering one of the 50 million soft drinks served in Disney World each year, why not make it interesting and drink it from a Test Track Cone or Chewbacca's head?

N

Naan

Nighttime Snacks

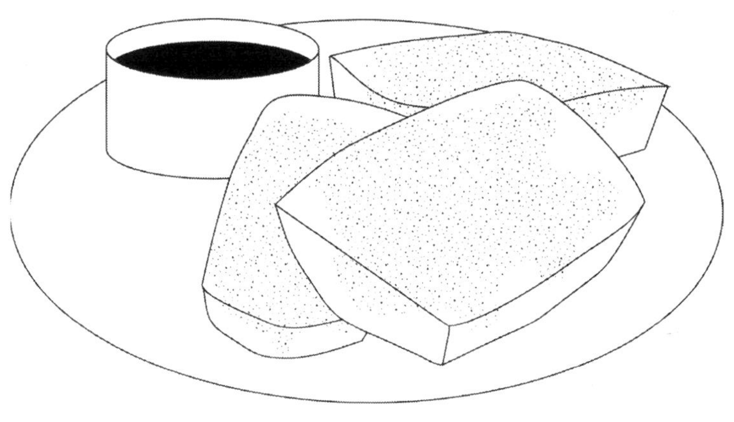

Naan

Naan has appeared and disappeared from festival and resort menus and the food trucks in Disney Springs, but it is always on the menu at Sanaa in Kidani Village at Animal Kingdom Lodge.

Naan is Indian-style bread that is a classy way to soak up sauces and curries. It is made by placing the dough on the inside of an incredibly hot tandoor, a clay oven that is actually on the ground or within a counter. Because of the high heat of the oven and the bread sticking to the wall of the tandoor as it cooks, the outside has a little crispiness, and is brown and soft on the inside with pockets of air that are perfect for scooping up delicious sauces. Naan is typically brushed with a bit of oil or butter.

The Indian-Style Bread Service is a must-have appetizer at Sanaa and offers a number of different breads, including traditional naan, spiced naan, and paneer paratha. The bread service comes with a wide selection of flavorful hummus, chutneys, jams, and dips. Our favorite chutneys were the mango and the coriander. The mango chutney has a bite to it and the coriander chutney has a brightness that was perfect with the paneer paratha. But the best way to have naan is dipped in the butter chicken sauce.

In 2015, we arrived at Disney World with only a few of our party of 11 ever having tasted naan. The chefs at Disney do naan so well we left with 11 naan-lovers all talking about going back to Disney, not to ride Tower of Terror, but to have that naan again.

Ordering Tip: Sanaa has a gluten-free menu that includes gluten-free naan.

Nighttime Snacks

Late-night snacks are available at most quick-service locations at the resorts and also at some lounges where they're available year-round, with most locations open until 11pm or midnight.

On an average day in the parks you will walk at least 5 miles. At the end of a 12-hour day a comfy resort bed sounds like the best option, but sometimes your stomach needs a bit of attention first. Nighttime snacks at a Disney resort come in a number of different shapes and sizes.

Many resorts offer some option to fulfill your late-night cravings. At the moderate resorts the food court is typically open late, until 11pm or midnight. Most moderate and value resorts and all deluxe resorts will also have a lounge that offers late-night treats. At deluxe resorts there is typically a table service or quick service open late and room service is also an option.

Most of the stores at the resorts will have snack sections. At villa resorts, the stores have small convenience store sections with options like frozen pizzas, macaroni and cheese, and Pop Tarts to make use of the stove, oven, or toaster in the room. These stores may not always be open that late, so plan accordingly.

With 23 resorts, all with different themes and foods to match, the nighttime snack offerings will keep you magically munching into the night. Here are five nighttime snacks not to be missed:

- Beignets from Sassagoula Float Works at Port Orleans French Quarter. This resort is a slice of Southern charm and is famous for beautiful grounds and enchanting fried dough. The beignets are copious and smothered in powdered sugar.
- Indian-Style Bread Service from Sanaa Lounge in Kidani Village at Animal Kingdom Lodge. Choose traditional naan for all three of the breads. Gorge and then head to bed full.
- Chips and dip from Rix Lounge at Coronado Springs. Have a new take on cookies and milk with chips and dip and a margarita flight. Nighttime never tasted so good.
- Late-night made-to-order pizza. These pizzas are available from quick-service locations at most resorts. Cheese, sausage and pepperoni are standard flavors. If you've been enjoying a bit of drinking at Disney, the pizza is the perfect way to absorb some of the alcohol. The pizzas are made to order, so be prepared to wait. Many resorts offer a call-ahead option.

 Gelato from Sassagoula Float Works. What is the perfect accompaniment to salty late-night pizza? A generous serving of gelato. There are multiple flavor options and the cast member behind the counter gave us an entire to-go container full of gelato. Not an ice cream container; the same to-go container as my individual pizza. That's a lot of gelato.

O

Ocean Beach Sea Salt Caramel Sundae

Outdoor Kitchens

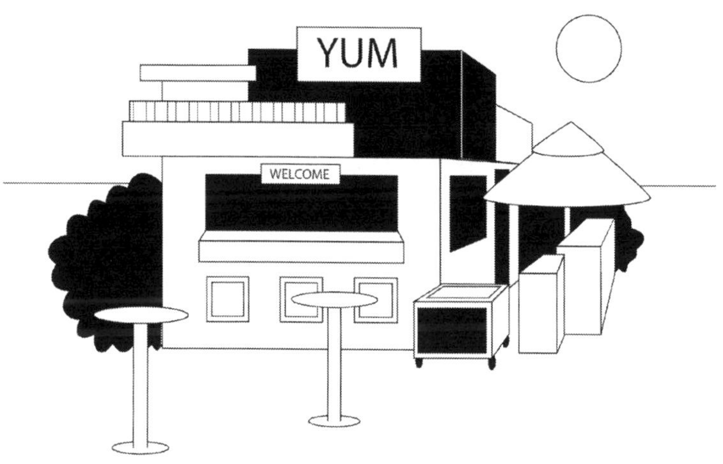

Ocean Beach Sea Salt Caramel Sundae

You'll find this decadent treat at Ghirardelli Ice Cream & Chocolate Shop at Disney Springs where it's available year-round. Have it as a late-night snack or as a late breakfast of champions. During most of the year, Ghirardelli's is open 10:30am to 11:30pm.

Location Tip: Free chocolate! Head into the chocolate-shop side of Ghirardelli's for a free sample.

You can smell Ghirardelli's before you see it. I think they may be pumping chocolate scent into the air. If you need your chocolate to-go, there is a small shop attached to the restaurant. Visiting Ghirardelli's is always on Austin's must-do list, along with scarfing down one of these sundaes. The Ocean Beach Sea Salt Caramel Sundae is vanilla ice cream with creamy caramel, hand-made hot fudge, and big chunks of sea salt. It's piled high with whipped cream, more crunchy sea salt, and a Ghirardelli chocolate square.

The sundae is huge and definitely sized (and priced) for sharing. It is very sweet—a bit too sweet for me. But for Austin: "This is as good as Starbucks. It's pricier, so I would hope it's better. It's a lot of salt at first. If you prefer a bit more sweet, you can ask them to add more caramel or cut back on the salt."

Ordering Tip: Order with a cup of ice water. The sundae can be pretty salty and the water helps.

Location Tip: Ghirardelli's has both indoor and outdoor seating. The outdoor area has comfortable tables and is a great place for people watching. During the holidays, there is a lovely view of festive decorations and the entrance to visit Santa.

Outdoor Kitchens

Outdoor Kitchens at the Epcot International Flower & Garden Festival feature farm-to-table food that focuses on fresh ingredients, often sourced locally. Whereas the Food Studios at Festival of the Arts have artistic plating, and Food & Wine is about trying new flavors, the dishes at the Outdoor Kitchens have a fresh and healthy feel—more like what would be on the table of a farmer who also happens to be a gourmet chef.

There are more dishes featuring fruits and vegetables here than at the other festivals. As a devout foodie, it's tough for me to say, but I like Flower & Garden more than Food & Wine. There are many more food options at Food & Wine, and then there is all the wine, but I prefer the style of food at Flower & Garden. And, as an added bonus, Epcot is at its most beautiful during this festival.

In 2017 there were 15 different Outdoor Kitchens, each typically offering 2-3 dishes and 4-5 beverage options. Like all things Disney, festival food changes every year. Some items like the watermelon salad and violet lemonade are classics that have staying power, but others don't stick around from year to year.

Every year the chefs from all the pavilion restaurants experiment in their own kitchens to determine what items will be on offer at the festivals. So, if Les Chefs de France is on your must-eat list, pop by the Fleur de Lys Outdoor Kitchen to see what Chef Bruno, the head chef of Les Chefs de France, has come up with. The good news: there will always be something new to try. The bad news: if you fall in love with a dish, say, the ratatouille tart at Fleur de Lys one year, when you go there again it may be gone. I had been thinking about that tart for four years since first having it in 2013. In 2017, no ratatouille tart. There was an onion tart, but it just wasn't the same.

Disney gives the Outdoor Kitchens flower-and-garden-sounding names. In 2017, they were:

- Urban Farm Eats served watermelon salad, a crabless cake, Wildflower Pale Ale, and the Urban Fairy Cocktail.
- Pineapple Promenade was a hot spot because it's one of the few places outside Magic Kingdom where you can find

Dole Whip, or as it's called at Flower & Garden, pineapple soft serve. A grown-up version with a shot of rum was also available. The other popular drink here is the photographically famous violet lemonade. Joe and I tried it and we're not fans. I would love to know how Disney is able to achieve the gorgeous purple of this drink, but, it looked better than it tasted. It was too sweet for us. The drink is sometimes served with an edible flower, but the violet lemonade is so popular that sometimes they run out of flowers. Pineapple Promenade also has a hot dog with pineapple chutney, but it's the drinks that draw a crowd.

- The Berry Basket, new in 2017, offered a lamb chop with blackberry gastrique and a field greens salad bursting with strawberries and blue cheese. But the highlight was a warm wild berry buckle with pepper berry sorbet. There was also a blueberry Moscato from a Florida vineyard to quench your thirst.
- La Isla Fresca featured dishes like Jamaican-braised beef, sugar cane shrimp skewers, and a FlanCocho for the sweet tooth. La Isla also had the famous Jamaican brew Red Stripe and a Frozen Simply Tropical Juice Drink served either grown-up style or booze-free for kids.
- Jardin de Fiestas in the Mexico Pavilion served up chile relleno de picadillo, a battered pepper with ground beef; tres leches, a traditional cake with three types of milk; and two flowery margaritas: hibiscus and elderflower.
- Lotus House, in China, had a spicy chicken lettuce wrap, Beijing-style candied strawberries, and a variety of fruity beverages like Oolong Peach Bubble Tea, Kung Fu Punch, and Dragon Pearl.
- Bauernmarkt: Farmer's Market, in Germany, offered potato pancakes with applesauce or topped with ham, onions, and herb sour cream. Flower & Garden fans washed down the currywurst and paprika chips with one of four beers, or sampled them all in a beer flight.
- Primavera Kitchen offered the fresh flavors of Italy. The antipasti misto was perfect for sharing, with six different

items on one plate, and at the other end of the meal, strawberry tiramisu. Italy offers 10 different ways to drink at Disney. The Rossini is a delicious blend of Prosecco (Italian sparkling wine) and marinated strawberries. If you fall in love with the Rossini, it's available at Tutto Gusto Wine Cellar even after the festival ends.

- American Adventure's Smokehouse was home to all the BBQ and brews, like pulled pig slider, smoked pork ribs, and beef brisket, with Shipyard Maple Bacon Stout or frozen lemonade with blackberry moonshine. For the kids: liquor-free frozen lemonade.
- Hanami, in Japan, offered one of the most interesting foods at Flower & Garden: fruishi, or fresh fruit sushi. Ahi tuna poke and beef teriyaki udon were also available. But really, everyone wants to try the fruishi just so you can say the word (and make a cast member say it). Hanami also offered two lagers and multiple sakes.
- Morocco's Taste of Marrakesh woke up some palates with a merguez "hot dog" sausage and house-made falafel. This kitchen also offered baklava and the beautiful Desert Rose cocktail.
- Florida Fresh, tucked between Morocco and France, was home to my second-favorite dish of Flower & Garden: shrimp and stone ground grits. The smooth creamy grits had whole kernels of corn for a nice crunch, and the shrimp on top was bursting with a bit of spiciness from the chorizo sausage and the freshness of the tomato. Together in one bite it was an explosion of flavors. We refreshed our palates for the next kitchen with a watermelon-cucumber slushy in virgin and non-virgin varieties, and local Florida beers.
- Fleur de Lys is near the fountain in France. Instead of the ratatouille tart, they had a Tarte l'Onion Alsacienne, an onion tart with thyme and rosemary, and a macaron chocolat framboise. The France Pavilion is well known for its macarons, and the La Vie en Rose Frozen Slush constantly receives votes for a favorite adult drink at the

festival. The brut de peche, a peach sparkling wine, paired beautifully with the macaron.

- Cider House in the UK was home to a number of tasty ways to fill your stomach—and get tipsy. The house-made potato and cheddar biscuit was a dish we polished off in a couple of bites. The biscuit had shreds of sharp cheddar cheese baked in, and was topped with fresh pink salmon, creamy mayo, and bright green dill. We cut the salt of the dish with the hard cider flight featuring black cherry, blood orange, and strawberry hard ciders. The black cherry is dangerously delicious with a tartness that cuts the sweetness of the cherry.
- Northern Bloom in Canada was another new addition in 2017. Festival foodies munched on seared scallops, beef tenderloin with bordelaise sauce, and a Nanaimo bar trifle while sitting next to the Bambi topiaries. The highlight from Canada was the maple popcorn shake. Joe and I tried it with a kick of Crown Royal and it seriously tastes like drinking maple popcorn. Make sure to grab a straw if you do it with the booze. The shot just sat on top of the milkshake. Without the straw and a quick stir, it was basically a seven-dollar shot of Crown Royal followed by a five-dollar milkshake.

The Outdoor Kitchens are a highlight of the Flower & Garden festival. The food and cocktails compliment the stunning flower displays and the aroma of fresh flowers and herbs that dance in the air throughout the park.

P

Paddlefish

Pool Bars

Popcorn

Pretzels, Mickey Shaped

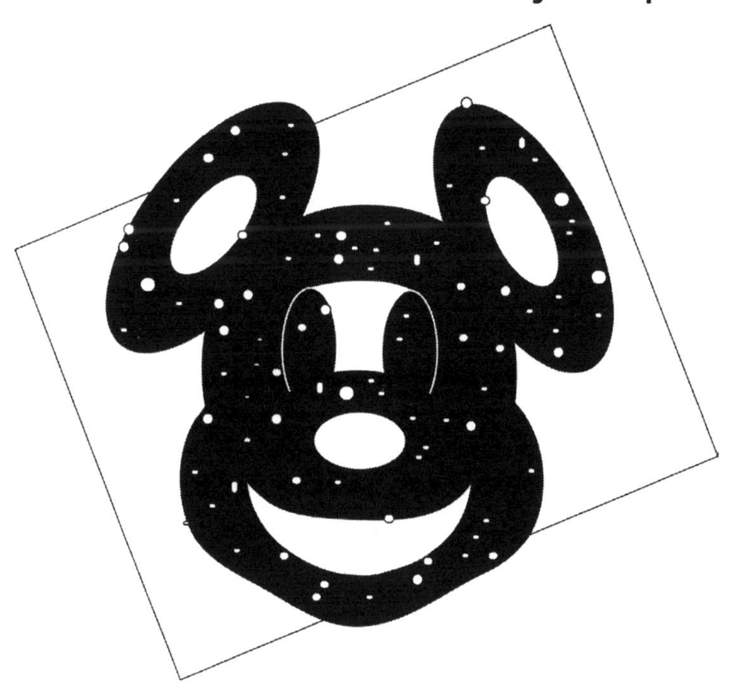

Paddlefish

Paddlefish, in The Landing at Disney Springs, is located on a big, multi-story boat and features seafood. No surprises there. But what is surprising is the novel way Paddlefish integrates seafood into corn dogs and guacamole.

There are oysters and crab legs a-plenty. Fried fish and clams galore. You want cocktails? They have plenty. But who cares? No big deal. I want *boils*. Ariel and Sebastian would hate this place! There are five different seafood boils, including a build-your-own, a full raw bar with oysters, shrimp, and ahi poke tuna.

Ordering Tip: With a large group that loves their fruits de mer (fruits of the sea), get the Seafood Tower. It's pricey but plentiful, and can check most of the traditional seafood boxes with jumbo Gulf shrimp, oysters, crab ceviche, tuna, and king crab.

Make sure to try the lobster corn dogs. The appetizer is beautifully plated with a generous piece of lobster on a skewer that is lightly fried in a sweet corn-dog batter. The lobster dogs are served with cabbage slaw and a sweet chili aioli for dipping. The sweetness of the corn batter plays up the natural butteriness in the lobster, and the sweet chili aioli adds a layer of heat and creaminess that I'm not sure is necessary. Definitely make sure to try it both ways, without aioli first.

In addition to a substantial selection of seafood, Paddlefish offers plenty of ambiance. There are three different dining rooms between the first and second floor, and two outdoor seating areas. The prime seating location is the plush couches and chairs on the top deck that offer a sweeping view of Disney Springs, the lake, and Saratoga Springs. This area is typically not open until the evening, but is worth a trip. The indoor spaces are nice, but it's the outdoor seating that is truly stunning. There is a second outdoor seating area on the first floor at the front of the restaurant and the space is beautiful. Boats and the Amphicars drift by. Birds chirp, and there is a relaxing sound from the tide lapping against the side of the boat. Since it's right on the open water, a gentle cooling breeze comes in. It really does feel like you're on a slow cruise on the water.

Location Tip: If it's August and miserably hot, a comfy deck seat may make for a sweaty, uncomfortable meal. But if it's spring or fall and early enough in the day, the outdoor seating area at the front of Paddlefish is the way to go.

In May 2017, Joe and I visited Paddlefish for an early lunch after a trip to the all-new Dress Shop at Cherry Tree Lane. This was just a quick stop for us to raise our blood sugar before diving into Epcot, so we kept things light with a crisp, cold glass of Pinot grigio for Joe and a bubbly Prosecco for me. For lunch we started with the lobster corn dog and, based on our waitress' recommendation, the crab cake. Both were light and delicious, but the true highlight of the meal was chatting with our waitress. This was our first Disney Springs dining experience and we were pleasantly surprised to receive the same passionate, high-quality Disney service that we've had while dining in the parks and resorts.

Pool Bars

Pool Bars are located at the main pool of many Disney resorts. Bigger resorts typically offer multiple pools, but one main themed-pool.

The pool bars all have fun names, like Petals at Pop Century, Turtle Shack at Old Key West, Leaping Horse at the BoardWalk Inn, Singing Spirits at All-Star Music, and Geyser Point at Wilderness Lodge.

At the value resorts, including Pop Century and Art of Animation, only grown-up libations and kid-friendly drinks are on the menu. Pop into the gift shop or have snacks for when the chlorine hits you and suddenly you're ravenous.

Moderate resorts vary in their pool bars. Port Orleans French Quarter is one of the smaller moderate hotels and pool guests can easily grab bites and drinks to go from Sassagoula Float Works. Coronado Springs is one of the largest moderate resorts and the pool is a hike from the main lobby and restaurant area. To make relaxing easier, the Siestas Cantina Pool Bar at Coronado Springs offers an extensive menu and even a breakfast with Mickey waffles. Eating a Mickey waffle by the pool? Now that is magical.

Deluxe resorts and most of the deluxe villa resorts offer a wide selection of libations and kid-friendly cocktails. Most also offer a pretty decent food menu and, like all things Disney, it is themed to the resort. So, while you can grab a chicken Caesar salad or lobster sliders at the Courtyard Pool Bar at Grand Floridian, if you're at the Maji Pool Bar at Kidani Village that Caesar Salad comes with tandoori chicken or the turkey sandwich has sambal mayo. Like all good Disney dining locations, the menus at the pool bars change regularly. You will always be able to get some sort of sandwich or salad or picnic-friendly food, but the pulled pork may not be available during your trip.

Disney gets why the grown-ups are there, and no matter which pool bar you visit, there is a wide selection of adult libation. A Sunken Treasure Cocktail at the Drop-Off Pool Bar at Art of Animation could help even Marlin from *Finding Nemo* calm down. A Frosty Pineapple at the Barefoot Pool Bar at the Polynesian Village features Dole Whip. Yes, Dole Whip in a cocktail form. A Passion Fruit Caipirinha or Coronado Crush will help with that afternoon nap at Siestas Cantina Pool Bar at Coronado Springs.

During our trip in 2015, Austin and I grabbed a late lunch of pulled pork sandwiches and chips at the Maji Pool Bar at Kidani Village. When you are swimming and starving everything tastes excellent, but that pulled pork was the perfect mix of tangy and sweet BBQ sauce. Maggie and I indulged in a few signature Disney cocktails. I'm not a fan of super-sweet cocktails and the piña-colada-inspired drink was definitely on the sweet side. But when you're sitting in the sunshine at a pool that resembles a watering hole in Africa, an icy tropical treat with hints of pineapple and coconut is apropos.

Popcorn

Popcorn at Disney just somehow tastes better. It must be the magical combination of butter and salt, but after a drop on Tower of Terror or during a parade on Main Street, few things are better than a bag of buttery, salty popcorn.

Popcorn is available throughout Disney World, and five million servings of popcorn are consumed there each year. Though most are eaten out of a typical Disney parks paper container, fun popcorn buckets are a big hit in the parks and shows the Disney merchandising machine at work.

Freshly popped corn at Disney World is primarily the butter-and-salt variety, but there are plenty of pre-bagged flavors that are made by the Main Street Popping Company and sold in Main Street Confectionery and at most stores throughout the parks and resorts. Even smaller stores, like the Frozen store outside the Frozen Sing-Along at Hollywood Studios, carry bags of popcorn. Some of the flavors include favorites like caramel, kettle corn, cheddar, or the brightly colored, sugary confetti corn, alongside more exotic flavors like sriracha kettle corn, parmesan garlic, churro, and maple bacon.

Location Tip: Head over toward the popcorn cart near the Figment attraction at Epcot to build your own festive popcorn mix for Halloween. On offer is bright yellow cheddar cheese, deep orange buffalo blue cheese, and a white sour cream and chive. Go crazy and ask them to do a mix of all three. It may look like traditional Halloween candy corn, but it's going to blow your mind with an explosion of spicy, cheesy, creamy, crunchy goodness.

From lotus flower buckets that light up for Rivers of Light and ornate Cinderella carriage buckets, to a Seven Dwarfs Mine Train cart, Disney has a popcorn bucket to meet all your popcorn storage needs. Cast member Nick remembers seeing a Stitch bucket designed so that Stitch's mouth held the popcorn: "You literally reach into his mouth to get the popcorn. You're eating popcorn from Stitch's mouth."

Nick is also a major Star Wars fan and loves the Tie-Fighter popcorn bucket: "This is a pretty massive contraption, but not the largest popcorn bucket, so you're basically carrying around this huge thing that only holds a small size popcorn." Star Wars fans also enjoy their popped corn out of the Darth

Vader bucket. Once again, you will be eating popcorn out of a character's head. Nick jokes, "Disney has a lot of head-shaped foods and buckets. Eating things out of a head is weird to me, but guests love them."

Pretzels, Mickey Shaped

Mickey pretzels are available throughout the four theme parks: look for the food carts that have a warmer on top. You can also find them at quite a few of the pool bars at Disney resorts. Mickey pretzels are available year-round, and are one of those Disney staples that with a little searching you can find almost anywhere.

The Mickey pretzel is yet another opportunity to eat your favorite mouse. The soft pretzel is shaped like Mickey's face and comes with a sprinkling of those big chunks of pretzel salt. The outside has a little bite to it and the inside is soft and chewy. Our favorite way to eat them is with the cheese sauce that comes in a cup for dipping.

These pretzels are the perfect on-the-go treat and make nighttime shows at Disney even more magical. In 2015, Annie and I were in charge of snacks and the one thing she had been wanting for three days was a Mickey pretzel. Her wish finally came true at Fantasmic. It's a bit disconcerting how many times a day we are gnawing on something shaped like our favorite mouse's head, but his ears dipped in a bit of cheese sauce was the perfect show-time snack.

A trip to Hollywood Studios isn't complete without a Mickey pretzel, even when we are at Disney without kids. In 2017, Joe and I grabbed a lunch of pretzels, cheese, and a seat just outside the Star Wars Launch Bay. We had a great view of Stormtroopers marching by as we munched on Mickey's face and licked liquid cheese off our fingers.

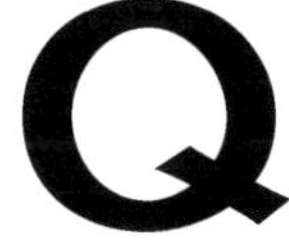

Queso Fundido
Quick Service

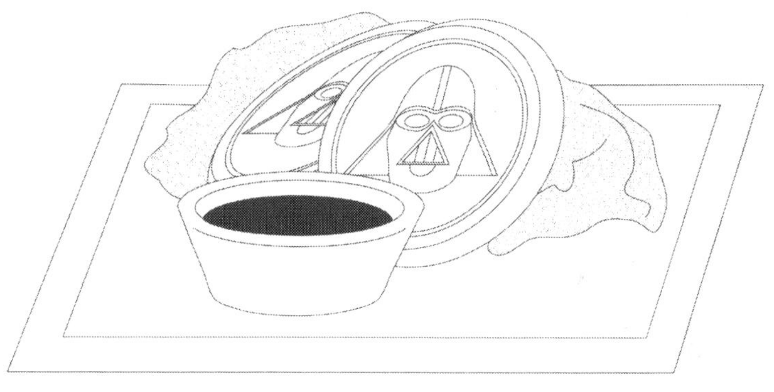

Queso Fundido

Queso fundido is available year-round at San Angel Inn in Epcot's Mexico Pavilion for lunch and dinner.

Ordering Tip: The queso is pretty filling. Make sure you either have a few folks to share it with or are famished after a day of Epcot walking.

San Angel Inn features up-scale Mexican food in one of the most beautiful and distinctive dining locations at Epcot, in the Mexico Pavilion. Austin and I visited San Angel in 2016. I ordered the queso fundido specifically to fulfill the letter Q, and am so glad I did. The dish arrives in a clay bowl with a wide opening for maximum dipping options. It is served with both flour tortillas and chips.

When it arrived Austin looked at it very skeptically and hesitantly dipped a tortilla chip. His eyes widened and he exclaimed, "Wow! This is delicious!" Austin is a fairly picky eater, and the last time I saw him enjoy a first bite this much it was a dish that involved a lot more sugar. The queso is gooey with the primary ingredient of salty melted cheeses. Chunks of spicy chorizo hide inside and give you a pop of spice when you catch one on your chip or tortilla. The queso is topped with poblano peppers that add a hit of sweetness and heat. It's an appetizing but filling way to start a meal at San Angel (and it pairs quite nicely with the jalapeno margarita).

Location Tip: The tables at San Angel are pretty close together. If you prefer to have more breathing room when eating, ask for a table on the water.

Quick Service

Quick-service locations can be found in every park, including the water parks, and at every resort (except some DVC locations).

Disney doesn't believe guests should have to compromise on quality when service is quick, and they've been working hard to make munching even more magical at quick-service and counter-service locations. Check out curry dogs at

Harambe Market at Animal Kingdom, fried shrimp or the lobster roll at Columbia Harbour House in Magic Kingdom, the Mediterranean falafel wrap at Tangierine Café in Morocco, a tartine aux fromages from Les Halles Boulangerie-Patisserie in France at Epcot, macaroni and cheese with pulled pork at Min and Bill's Dockside Diner in Hollywood Studios, or a quick Mickey ice cream bar just about anywhere.

Quick-Service Tip: Many quick-service locations offer seating either at the location or nearby. For large and busy venues with seating, split up. Have one person take the order while another finds a table. For locations without seating, have one person find seating before you are balancing a heavy tray with a trough of fries, ginormous hot dogs, and vats of soda.

Here are some quick-service favorites from taste testers and cast members alike:

- **Harambe Market, Africa, Animal Kingdom.** Cast member Nick "really likes Harambe Market for quick service. It has some of the most unique food. The ribs are exotic and have an African spice with warm flavors and smoke."
- **Be Our Guest, Fantasyland, Magic Kingdom.** It feels weird to call Be Our Guest quick service, as it has some of the best food in all of Magic Kingdom. But, for breakfast and lunch it *is* quick service. Though enchanting, it is not the quickest, but it has the grey stuff and it's delicious.
- **Food Kiosks at Epcot Festivals.** Over 196 different dishes from 20 different countries at four festivals. That's a lot of quick, magical bites.
- **Les Halles Boulangerie & Patisserie, France Pavilion, Epcot.** Many delicious quick-service locations are dotted around World Showcase. Because all of the table-service locations are so delicious, and talking with the cast members who work at them is one of our favorite things to do, we just don't visit a lot of Epcot quick service. Les Halles is a place we do love to go for breakfast

and it is open before most of the other World Showcase restaurants. And it's home to macarons as well.

- **Colombia Harbour House, Liberty Square, Magic Kingdom.** The fried shrimp. That's all you need to know. Order the fried shrimp.
- **Pepper Market, Coronado Spring Resort.** Empanadas, black beans, yogurt parfaits, and Chef Vance are just a few of the many reasons this one is on our list.
- **Morimoto Street Food at Disney Springs.** Nick visits this spot for quick bites of bao, sushi, and dumplings. It's a great lunch spot and has covered seating overlooking a small, bright blue pond.
- **Mr Kamal's, Asia, Animal Kingdom.** This is Chef Lee's favorite place in all of Disney World. "The fresh falafel pitas are so amazing and so good. On my days off I would go to Animal Kingdom just to get that. It was cheap and delicious. I would fly from Chicago now to go there."
- **Backlot Express at Hollywood Studios.** Until the new Star Wars Land opens, this is the home of Star Wars-themed food. Darth Vader chicken and waffles are a must for any Star Wars fan.
- **Disney Food Trucks at Disney Springs.** Mallorie from Le Chefs de France visits the Food Trucks because "they are affordable and you can try many different things." The food trucks can be pretty elusive and have very specific hours. If you're looking for a delicious snack at 10pm and are in the right Disney Springs spot at the right time, you may just get lucky and try some of the classic items these food trucks serve.

R

Restaurant Marrakesh
Roast Beef
Room Service

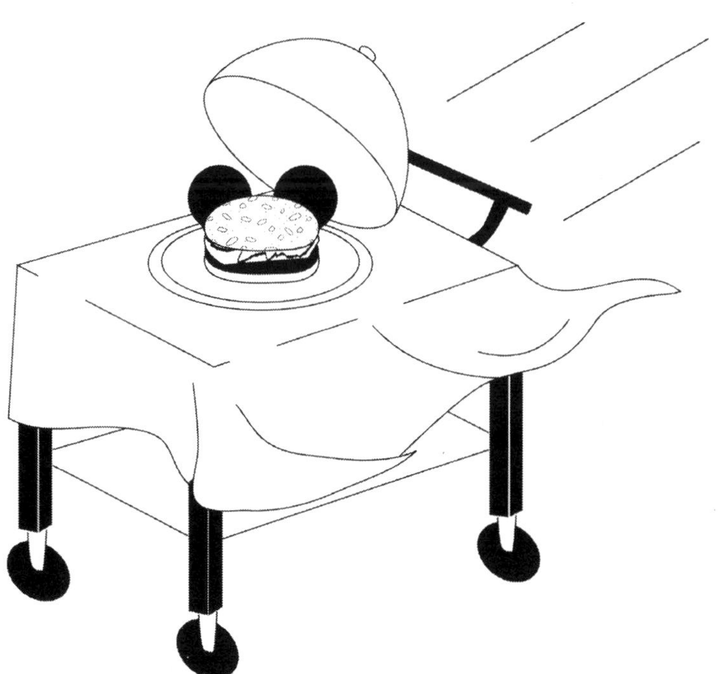

Restaurant Marrakesh

Restaurant Marrakesh is in the Morocco Pavilion at Epcot. To find it, you have to journey into the depths of the pavilion. This has helped it remain a hidden gem that is one of the best-themed, most authentic World Showcase restaurants that most guests have never been to.

The dinner and lunch menus are different. We recommend going for lunch. The menu has more traditional Moroccan dishes that combine meats with warm spices and sweet toppings like cinnamon, powdered sugar, and almonds. This is not the tourist version of Moroccan food.

Make sure to try the appetizer combo: beef brewat rolls, chicken bastilla, and jasmina salad. You'll get many of the most exotic tastes on the menu on one plate.

After checking in, you enter through an ornately decorated lobby area, then you are taken into a grand ballroom with soaring ceilings and tiled pillars where you are greeted by live musicians playing authentic Moroccan music. It feels like you are in the heart of a royal palace. And the smells. Meats roasting in cinnamon and spices, rice flavored with curry and dried fruits, and the sweet smells of phyllo dough mixed with powdered sugar and almonds.

Location Tip: To have the best view of the band and the belly dancer, ask to sit toward the center of the restaurant.

Adding to the ambiance is the live band and the beautiful belly dancer. What was truly entertaining during our visit in 2005 was watching 5-year-old Austin watching the belly dancer. He was initially sitting with his back to her, but upon discovering her presence and dancing ability, he sat enthralled with his back turned to us during her entire performance. He kept eating, though, not once turning around and just reaching back to grab his bites. Discovering your child's love of belly dancing and your family's love of cinnamon-spiced meat—just another magical day at Epcot.

Roast Beef

Roast beef is served at Be Our Guest in Magic Kingdom ... sometimes. The carved prime chuck roast beef sandwich had been on the lunch menu since 2013 and is one of Joe's favorite foods at Disney. It has been replaced by another sandwich, the French Dip. This still has roasted beef, just sliced a bit thinner. It's another lesson in Disney dining and the danger of liking something a bit too much.

There are many similarities between the two sandwiches. Both are served on a warm baguette. Both have tender roast beef, lightly seasoned. Both are served with thin, crispy pomme frites (French fries). One big difference is that the previous roast beef sandwich was served with a horseradish sour cream to add a bit of heat and was topped with peppery arugula.

Some of our other favorites, like the smooth, creamy potato leek soup, are still on the menu. When our group of 11 were at Be Our Guest in 2015, half of us ordered the braised pork cooked coq au vin style. The pork is served with mashed potatoes and vegetables. The croque monsieur is a French version of grilled cheese. Gruyere cheese and béchamel sauce combine to make a rich sauce that rests on top of the carved ham and is soaked into the crusty baguette.

Despite removing Joe's favorite sandwich from the menu, Be Our Guest is still magical and our favorite restaurant at Magic Kingdom. Just do me a solid, Disney chefs, and please keep the Grey Stuff!

Room Service

After a long day at the parks, room service can be a godsend. It's important to note that not all Disney World resorts have room service, but resorts in the deluxe and villas categories usually do. At press time, only Coronado Springs among the moderates offered room service.

At the deluxe and villas resorts, room service is incredible and can be on par with the restaurants themselves. Like everything else at Disney, room service is themed to the resort. They all have a standard and kids menu and must-have room service items like burgers and basic sandwiches, as well as unique items that match the theme of the resort. At Wilderness Lodge you can get a grilled northwest chicken sandwich or wilderness salad. The Polynesian has multiple seafood options and even in-room sushi. Head to Animal Kingdom Lodge and Kidani Village for exotic items like naan and tandoori chicken.

In 2015, after a travel day that started at 3am and a few hours in Magic Kingdom, the room service at Kidani Village did the trick to put us all to sleep. As *Monsters University* played in the background, Nate, Austin, and Nickolas chowed down on burgers and naan.

Room Service Tip: Plan ahead when ordering. Disney resorts are massive. At around 8:30am there may be a few hundred people craving bacon and eggs from room service. This means the wait for can be lengthy. If possible, order when other guests are *not* ordering.

At Kidani Village in 2015 I was craving a Midwestern breakfast of bacon, eggs, and carb-loading. After waiting on hold with room service for 10 minutes and then finding out that it was a minimum 45-minute wait on top of that, I grabbed a donut and hit the parks. It's not the right way to start a day. The only cure was a vat of Coca-Cola and riding Expedition Everest two times in a row. The great news? Sanaa, the restaurant at Kidani Village, now serves breakfast.

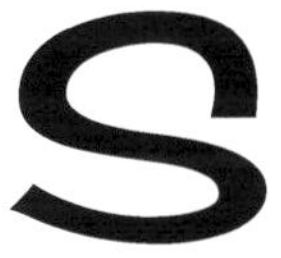

Sanaa

San Angel Inn

Sci-Fi Dine-In Theatre

Spice Road Table

Starbucks

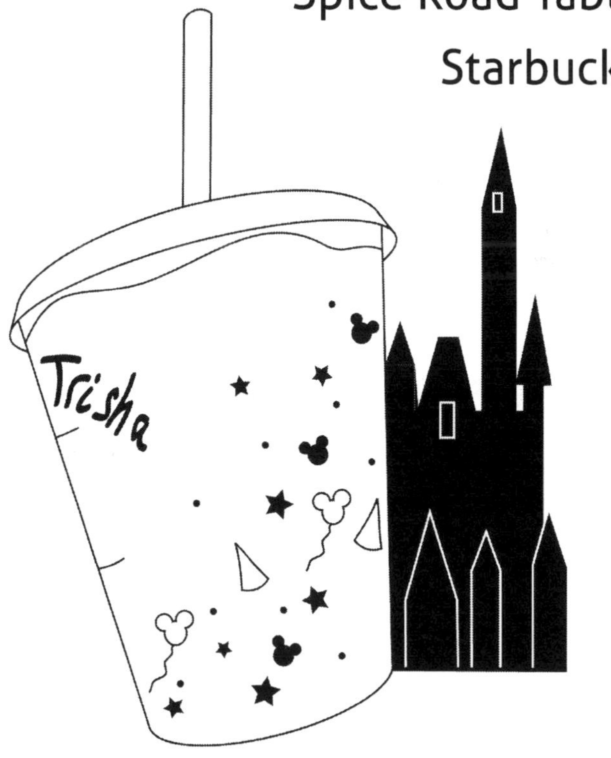

Sanaa

Sanaa, at Kidani Village at Animal Kingdom Lodge, serves African food with Indian flavors sprinkled in. The interior of Sanaa is beautiful, with dark wood tables, colorful walls, and arched windows. What is truly spectacular is the location —right on the savannah. Large windows throughout the restaurant put you right in the action with giraffes, zebras, gazelles, wildebeests, and many of the over 30 species of animals calling the four savannahs home. The animals are not shy and will often come close enough to the restaurant that you can see the giraffes long tongues grabbing at food.

Location Tip: Kidani Village and Animal Kingdom Lodge are not in the same building. They are about a mile apart. At most parks and at Disney Springs there is a bus listed specifically for Kidani Village. If there is not, take the bus to the lodge, but let the driver know you need to go to Kidani Village.

Sanaa is open for breakfast, lunch, and dinner. It is growing in popularity, so reservations are recommended. Sanaa Lounge serves appetizers and cocktails. The lunch and dinner menus are slightly different, though the Indian-Style Bread Service and Potjie-Inspired are served at both.

Make sure to try the Butter Chicken and the Indian-Style Bread Service appetizer. The Painted Lemur cocktail is playful and served in a glass with chocolate-stripes inspired by its namesake.

Ordering Tip: Sanaa has a gluten-free and allergy menu. Just ask.

Lunch is our preferred meal at Sanaa. Our group of 11 chose it twice on our trip in 2015. Austin and I had been dreaming about the butter chicken for a year, so we went again for lunch in 2016. Sunset is also a nice time to visit, as the animals are active. The path to their bed is right in front of the restaurant and seeing them all making the trek is fascinating. It's like being in the opening scene of *The Lion King*. But without the lions, because that might be bad...

Location Tip: When checking in, ask to be seated near a window. That way a zebra can stand there and watch you munch on your Spice Trade candy bar while a group of gazelles play tag in the distance.

San Angel Inn

San Angel Inn is at Epcot's Mexico pavilion. There are two other restaurants in the Mexico pavilion with San Angel in the name. San Angel Inn is the only restaurant inside the pyramid. Next door is a small tequila bar called La Cava del Tequila. San Angel Inn is modeled after a 17th century hacienda, so diners feel as if they are sitting outdoors.

Location Tip: When checking in, ask to sit along the water. It's such a beautiful place to dine with the dark blue sky overhead and the boats going by on the inky black water. You can even hear the water gently lapping against the edge of the restaurant.

Some dishes at San Angel Inn have a more Mexican-American feel, while others, like the Mole Poblano, which features chicken in a mole sauce, are more authentic.

Ordering Tip: The menu changes regularly. Some items, like the queso fundido and the tacos, are pretty standard, but if you find something you like while there, eat a lot. It may be gone next time.

This happened to me during our May 2017 trip. I had been craving the Tostadas de Tinga I enjoyed during a trip just five months prior, but they were no longer on the menu. I drowned my sorrows in a margarita flight and chips and guacamole. The guacamole was smooth with little bursts of sweet juice from pomegranate seeds, and served with a generous helping of red sauce to add a kick. If you prefer mild, make sure to ask for the red sauce on the side. The chips we received were not traditional flour or corn tortilla chips; they were super-crunchy corn cones, similar to Bugles, except a very high-end type of Bugles. The chips were airy and the crunch provided a nice texture contrast to the smooth guacamole.

Ordering Tip: The margarita flight is not on the menu, but ask politely and your server may hook you up. This is a fun way to try some of the many flavors of margarita served at La Cava del Tequila.

Location Tip: San Angel can have pretty tight quarters, with many tables in a small space. This may mean you are sitting fairly close to guests at the next table. Along the water or walls the tables have a bit more space. Also, with the dark sky and low table lighting, it can also be fairly dark. With my old eyes, I always have to use my cell phone to read the menu.

San Angel Inn is one of the most romantic restaurants in Disney World, especially if you can sit along the water. It is also popular for birthdays. During our last trip, there were three guests treated to a song and a treat. This is also a great place to take teens and grown-ups who are picky eaters but want to have a unique/themed dining experience in World Showcase. There are some familiar favorites on the menu, but the ambiance is nothing like the Taco Bell back home.

Sci-Fi Dine-In Theatre

Sci-Fi Dine-In Theatre is off Commissary Lane at Hollywood Studios. Stepping inside is like going back in time to a 1950s drive-in theatre. It's a big dark room with walls painted to look like a neighborhood, complete with glowing windows on houses. At the end of the block there is a giant movie screen. Diners sit facing the screen in old cars that have been converted into booths. There are café-style tables along the outer edge and the kitchen looks like a concession stand.

Sci-Fi's menu is in keeping with the 1950s diner theme: burgers, shakes, and a few pastas and salads thrown in, just in case. The burgers are gigantic, the fries crispy, and the shakes thick and creamy. They even have cocktails for the grown-ups.

Location Tip: Ask to sit in a car when you check in. Sitting in the cars while watching the old movies really makes the experience.

During the meal, Sci-Fi entertains with trailers of cheesy old science-fiction movies including Oliver's favorite *Attack of the 50-Foot Woman*. Sci-Fi is Nate's favorite restaurant at Disney World and it's always on our list. In 2015, Annie discovered another Sci-Fi perk: it's a good place to take a quick nap. I almost joined her after a few sips of the Habanero Lime Martian Margarita. It was just what the Disney doctor ordered. Sci-Fi servings are *very* generous. Unless you're starving, you can probably get away with sharing. There are a lot of options on the menu: New York strip, pastas, and a caprese sandwich. The onion rings are a must. They are always straight from the fryer, so the outside is crisp, the onions are sweet, and they taste great with a quick dip in a pool of ketchup.

Ordering Tip: One special treat that can be a fun souvenir item are light-up cups. These are just standard Disney cups that have a plastic character or symbol with a light inside (some of them clip on and others are used like ice cubes). The Disney marketing machine is in full force with these cups and they are always themed to the latest movie, show, or big event. At past Star Wars weekends there were light-up Death Stars added to the strawberry lemonade. One of Oliver's most memorable light-up cups was Lightning McQueen at Sci-Fi. It's pretty cool to order a light-up cup at a dark restaurant because you can see your cup glowing from across the room long before it reaches your table. It just increases the anticipation for your little one ... and helps you feel a bit better about the cost of this pricey souvenir.

Make sure to try the milk shakes. Just like at any 50s diner, the shakes are thick and fattening and served in a frosty glass. Ask about that day's specialty flavor. Also ask about the seasonal specialty burger.

Spice Road Table

Spice Road Table, in Epcot's Morocco Pavilion, is aptly named for its menu of bold, spicy Mediterranean flavors. There are a number of small-plate options. The three lamb sliders—almost like Moroccan tapas, mixed grill skewers, and the Mediterranean vegetable platter entrees are all of shareable size.

In the beverage department, you'll find a selection of Mediterranean beers from Morocco, Turkey, and even Lebanon. The cocktail menu has a few options not found at many other restaurants.

Spice Road Table is gorgeous. Its location right on the Seven Seas Lagoon gives it a stunning view of Spaceship Earth and the World Showcase. There is both indoor and outdoor seating. The inside of the restaurant has large windows looking out on the lagoon with ornate furniture and deep cerulean walls in the bar area. The light fixtures with different colored glass cast a romantic glow over both the indoor and outdoor spaces.

Outside is a tiled, covered patio with cushioned metal chairs. In the outdoor area you have your choice of two views. One side is perfect for people watching, as it's right on the main World Showcase drag. You can even hear the lively and energetic band that plays in the Morocco Pavilion. The other side looks out onto the lagoon with friendly ducks and World Showcase spread out on either side.

Location Tip: Make sure you have an extra layer of clothing with you. The lagoon can kick up some wind. We were there on a day that was well over 90 degrees, and Joe and I were both chilly as the sun went down.

Joe and I had a table for two outside at Spice Road during our trip in 2017. We stuck to all shareable small plates: lamb sausage, harissa chicken roll, spicy garlic shrimp, and two rounds of hummus fries. All of the dishes were packed with flavor and a fiery bit of heat.

Two must-try items are the hummus fries and the Marbella Summer cocktail. The fries are crispy on the outside and creamy on the inside with heat and a depth of flavor added by the harissa sauce. The Marbella Summer cocktail looks like an intense sunset in a glass. It's served frozen and has strawberries with brandy and Gran Gala liqueur.

Ordering Tip: Florida heat is the perfect excuse to drink a cocktail quickly. I learned the hard way that the Marbella Summer is better when it's still frozen (though it was a perfect excuse to order another).

The most magical part of most World Showcase restaurants is talking with the servers and other cast members. Our server was from Casablanca. He shared stories of growing up in Morocco and how his mother used to make her own bread dough at home. His mother would then send him to the baker to have the bread baked. He shared that the bread served at Spice Road Table reminds him of the one he would carry home from the baker.

Location Tip: Make a reservation for around 8pm and request to sit outdoors. Spice Road Table offers an amazing view for IllumiNations. There are plenty of magical views for IllumiNations, but the one at Spice Road Table comes with a seat, and food, and tasty drinks.

Starbucks

If Starbucks is a necessary part of your morning routine, Disney has you covered. The four theme parks and Disney Springs each have at least one Starbucks.

Location Tip: Most of the Starbucks are so busy they have two lines. At the location in

Epcot's Future World, the line to the right is often overlooked and much shorter. Once we were able to basically walk up to the pastry counter. Be prepared to get dirty looks from guests standing in the line to the left.

There are even special Disney Starbucks cups with stars and castles and the Disney logo. But what makes the Starbucks really Disney-esque is cast members like Josh, who works at the Starbucks in Disney Springs. Josh is like the barista you have back home who always greets you with a smile. With the castle drawn onto his name badge, a Santa hat during the holidays, and a magical grin, Josh has all the qualities we love in Disney cast members, but with the mad Frappuccino-making skills of the best Starbucks barista.

Ordering Tip: Starbucks in the Disney parks do not have bagels. If a bagel is what gets you up in the morning, pop over to a quick-service location at a resort. If it must be a bagel of the Starbucks variety, it's off to Disney Springs with you. They have bagels there.

Most of the Disney Starbucks have the standard set of pastries found at most Starbucks, including Austin's favorite, the bacon, egg, and gouda. Since it is Disney, there are a few Disney-specific pastry items, like a chocolate cupcake with chocolate cookie Mickey ears and a Frozen cupcake.

They also have holiday specific treats like the peppermint crunch cupcake. This cupcake was all about the looks, and was not so good. It was a chocolate cake with a bright red peppermint frosting topped with a candy cane. The cupcake was a pricey disappointment, overly sweet and bitter because of the red dye used to make the frosting a bright Christmas red.

If you are in the mood for sweets, walk a few doors down to the Main Street Confectionery. The pastries are a bit fresher and have a better balance of flavors.

T

Tacos

Tiffins

Tune-In Lounge

Tutto Gusto Wine Cellar

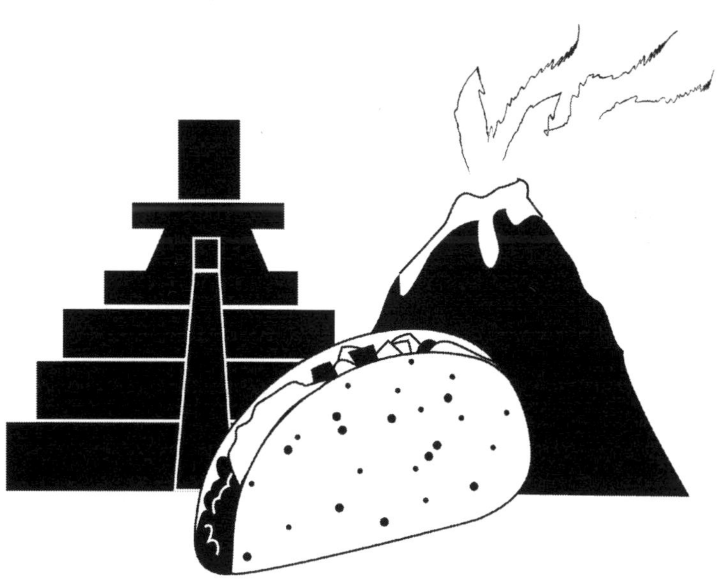

Tacos

I love tacos. A shrimp taco with lime sour cream and chunks of avocado makes a perfect lunch on a summer day. Walking tacos in a bag of nacho cheese Doritos are perfect at a chilly fall game. The perfect hangover prevention food? Taco Bell. I couldn't do a book about food without a little taco love.

Disney loves tacos, too. Maybe not as much as turkey legs or Mickey ice cream, but some magical tacos can be found at Disney World:

- *Festival tacos at Food & Wine Festival at Epcot.* The tacos in Mexico at Food & Wine may be small, but they are mighty on flavor.
- *Late-night tacos at the Springs Street Taco Food Truck at Disney Springs.* Pork belly or grilled steak are best for staving off a hangover. Can't decide? Get a Taco Combo.
- *Tacos with the best view are at San Angel Inn in Epcot.* The menu changes, but there are always taco appetizers or entrees. The tacos vegetales are messy but delicious.
- *Tacos to go at Pepper Market at Coronado Springs.* At Pepper Market you can build your own tacos. Don't forget the scrumptious black beans.
- *Artsy tacos at El Artista Hambriento at Epcot's Festival of the Arts.* This is the letter C taco trifecta: corn tortillas, chorizo, and chihuahua cheese.
- *Storytelling tacos at Nomad Lounge in Animal Kingdom.* Every drink and dish at Nomad Lounge has a story of the adventures that inspired it.

If a week at Disney without tacos sounds as crazy as a day without Starbucks, visit one of the tasty taco options above, or seek out your own. There are over 30 places at Disney World to get your taco on.

Tiffins

Tiffins is in the Discovery Island area of Animal Kingdom, right near Pandora. It is a gourmet restaurant with a story and cuisine inspired by the extensive and exotic travels of Disney Imagineer Joe Rohde, the man behind much of what you see at Animal Kingdom. The restaurant is a tribute to all of the adventures Joe and his team undertook to create the park.

Tiffins is a foodie paradise, with flavors from far-off places like Africa, India, Peru, and the Middle East. Dishes range from black-eyed pea fritters and roasted vegetable curry to calamansi mousse. It is for the adventurous eater; a cheeseburger cannot be found on the menu. But a meal here is like no other at a Disney park. You will be transported to another world, so take a culinary risk and have a meal you will not forget.

Location Tip: There are three dining rooms at Tiffins: the Grand Gallery, the Safari Gallery, and the Trek Gallery. The largest is the Grand Gallery. The Trek Gallery is off the Nomad Lounge and has big picture windows, so ask for this space if you prefer sunlight. If you have an animal lover in your group, go for the Grand Gallery; it features artwork and Rivers of Light-inspired illuminated installations everywhere you turn. It is especially stunning at night. Make sure to visit every room before leaving and, if possible, ask a cast member to tell you the story of each.

Location Tip #2: If you crave Animal Kingdom nostalgia and miss Camp Mickey and Minnie, make sure to stop in the Grand Gallery. Disney salvaged a few of the totem poles from Camp Mickey and Minnie and had the roof of Tiffins raised so that these relics could be placed in the Grand Gallery.

The quality ingredients, gorgeous plating, exotic flavors, and impeccable service will make you forget you are even at a theme park. In 2017, my husband Joe and I had a grown-ups-only trip to Disney, and dinner at Tiffins was the highlight of an entire trip devoted to food. Our meal started with a Snow Leopard Cocktail for me, and a Kungaloosh beer for Joe. Kungaloosh is Disney's own beer. A Disney first! The cocktails are served in stunning glassware with the signature paper straws of Animal Kingdom. Our server, Allie, was on the opening team of the restaurant and her passion and extensive knowledge of the dishes, chef, and story of the Tiffins entertained us throughout our multi-course dinner.

Ordering Tip: The menu is always changing and focuses on the freshest ingredients of the season. The most up-to-date menu is posted outside the restaurant. Joe and I experienced a spring-inspired menu during our trip in May.

The menu is the same for lunch and dinner, and features an extensive selection of appetizers. We splurge for the marinated grilled octopus and Tiffins' signature bread service for Joe, and the lobster-popcorn Thai curry soup and sustainable fish causa for me. Chefs will say you eat with your eyes and nose first, and the plating of these four appetizers was art. The soup comes in a crisp white bowl that highlights the small scoops of lobster popcorn. A server then comes and slowly pours in the broth. Immediately the smells of subtle curry, buttery lobster, and just a hint of lemongrass hit you. There are so many layers of flavor in this soup that the more you eat, the more you taste. Make sure to join the clean plate club so you don't miss any of the lobster popcorn hiding at the bottom of the bowl. Those little nuggets of buttery goodness explode on your tongue.

Ordering Tip: Order the bread service to soak up all the sauces in your appetizers and entrees. It's served in a beautiful, silver-tiered container, sometimes called a tiffin, which is the word used for a light midday lunch in India, and is the restaurant's namesake. The bread service tiffin contains different breads and sauces like black pea hummus, a spicy Indian-style salsa, and zough yogurt for dipping. Our service included papadum, a thin crispy chip, almost like a tortilla chip, with a touch of curry salt. The papadum was perfect to dip in my soup. The roti, a flatbread similar to naan, was the perfect way to soak up all the delicious bits of soup that my spoon couldn't reach. Joe used it to finish off the saffron aioli in his marinated grilled octopus.

For our entrées, Joe ordered the pan-seared duck breast with parsnip puree, truffle reduction, and huckleberry compote. The duck was perfectly cooked, with a crispy skin and meat that melted in his mouth. The plate also included beautiful thin mushrooms.

Though Joe's dish won in taste, my duo of venison won the plating award. The venison comes as medallions and sausages on a bed of different sauces and seasonings, including chakalaka. Take a moment and say that word. It's as fun to eat as it is to say. It means something with two ingredients. On this day it was tomato and onions. The dish was served on a white plate, occupying just a quarter of the plate with a sprinkling of leek ash on the edge. The effect is stunning. It is reminiscent of the black-and-white cookie, but in place of black frosting, you have meat and leek ash on a sharp white plate.

For dessert I went with savory and the assortment of artisanal cheeses. This was the salty that paired beautifully with Joe's sweet South American chocolate ganache. Joe also tried the Mustang Coffee (pronounced Moo-stang, after the coffee Joe Rohde was served in Mustang, Nepal), which contains butter, brown sugar, and Crown Royal. We never would have thought to put butter in coffee but it has since been an experiment at home. The cheese plate is a creamy array of different soft, semi-soft, and hard cheeses served with fig and anise bread, fig cake, passion fruit jelly, and local honey. A dollop of honey with a smear of the semi-soft Brie on the chewy, slightly bitter fig and anise bread was a perfect blend of textures and flavors.

Dining Package Tip: If you are doing the Rivers of Light dining package, you must order an appetizer, entrée, and dessert. You can always order more of any course, like we did with the

appetizers. You can also have the assortment of artisanal cheeses in place of something sweet.

Tiffins is a journey for all of your senses, from the stunning plating and brightly colored art adorning the walls, the cast member stories, the smells of curry mingling with fruits and game, the heavy flatware and soft curves of the cocktails glasses, to the flavors that burst on your tongue. This restaurant is a showpiece of Disney Imagineering at its best. What does one do after a gourmet meal in a theme park? Ride a roller coaster, of course. In tribute to all the creativity and sense of adventure of Joe Rohde and the Imagineers, we trekked with our full bellies to Asia and rode Expedition Everest. Twice.

Tune-In Lounge

Tune-In Lounge is at Hollywood Studios, right off Echo Lake and next to the 50's Prime-Time Café. It pulls from the café menu and features good, old-fashioned comfort food that you'd find on the dinner table of a 1950s suburban family home. You can tuck into all the classics of the 50s like fried chicken, meatloaf, mashed potatoes, and even chicken pot pie.

Tune-In Lounge is an eclectically decorated space that feels more like a room in your grandparent's house, or sitting in a Technicolor episode of *Leave It to Beaver.* Reservations aren't required for the lounge, but getting a seat can be tricky. It is a popular hangout for guests in the know.

As a tribute to all the dads back in the 50s who actually ventured into the kitchen, make sure you try Dad's Electric Lemonade and Grandpa's Crab Cake.

Most folks just come in to wait for their café reservation, but we started a trend during our 2013 trip by taking a seat on a pastel-colored leather couch in front of an old black-and-white TV and enjoyed a tray of comfort food right there in the lounge. Oliver munched on cheese, grapes, and a smoothie, while Joe and I shared A Sampling of Mom's Favorites. Sitting on a lime green sofa eating crispy fried chicken with creamy mashed potatoes and sipping Dad's Electric Lemonade while watching some black-and white TV shows felt very 50s indeed.

Tutto Gusto Wine Cellar

Tutto Gusto Wine Cellar is a lounge in Epcot's Italy Pavilion. It's easy to miss, as it's tucked away next to Tutto Italia restaurant.

Location Tip: Ask the host or hostess if you can sit near the fireplace. It's a beautiful, intimate space and we always make friends with other guests whenever we sit there.

Tutto Gusto Wine Cellar has a full menu of Italian fare but specializes in small plates. Make sure to try a meat-and-cheese plate with creamy mozzarella, salty prosciutto, and finocchiona—a salami flavored with fennel and black pepper. The perfect accompaniment is the fruity sparkling Rossini, a cocktail with fresh strawberry puree and a light bubbly Prosecco. It's like summer in a glass.

Epcot is jam-packed with amazing restaurants, and with so many choices there are a number of delightful hidden gems. While most people head to the full-service and larger Tutto Italia restaurant, we prefer the smaller, more intimate Tutto Gusto Wine Cellar. Any restaurant with "wine cellar" in the name gets our attention.

Tutto Gusto provides a sanctuary from the heat with its brick walls and eclectic light fixtures. They keep the door open so you aren't blasted by the Florida air conditioning. Our trip in 2017 was our second visit to Tutto Gusto and was just as lovely as the first one. We had a little table in front of a fireplace and sat on an overstuffed couch with a coffee table in front of us.

The wait staff is all from Italy and we met the lovely Nicoletta, who entertained us with stories from her village and her Papa's take on American-Italian food. She told us: "My favorite dish is the lasagna. When guests order it, I love to tell them the story of the plate and where it came from in Italy. I want to give every guest a magical Italian moment."

U

Unique Eats
Urban Fairy Cocktail

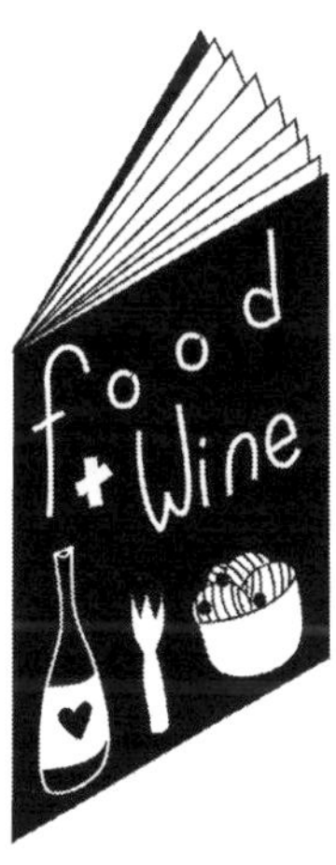

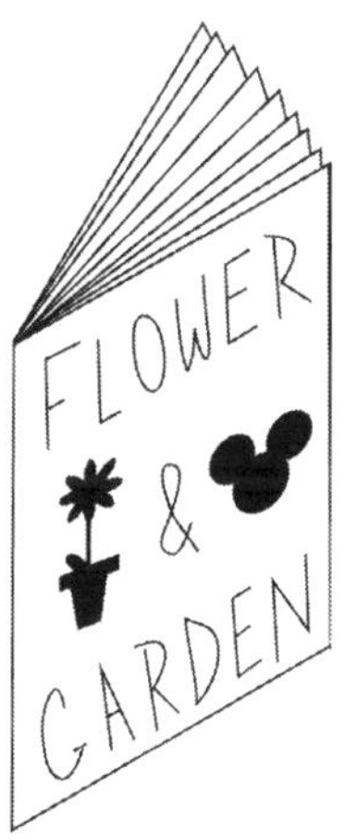

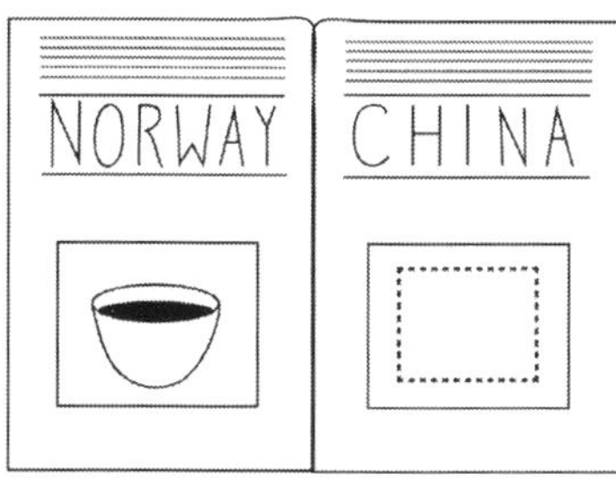

Unique Eats

Harissa chicken roll, Three Kings bread, Mickey and Pluto white chocolate painting with chocolate easel, and Violet Lemonade with fresh edible flowers. Any of these sound intriguing? Then you should visit Epcot during one of the its four foodie-friendly festivals.

Every Epcot festival features magical experiences, world-class entertainment, special events, education courses, and of course, food! Our favorite part of any Epcot fest is the selection of food and beverages at kiosks dotted around Future World and World Showcase. Each festival has a different name for the must-visit food kiosks.

As of 2017, Epcot is home to four different festivals featuring delicious food options: Epcot International Festival of the Arts, Epcot International Flower & Garden Festival, Epcot International Food & Wine Festival, and Epcot International Festival of the Holidays.

Between the four festivals almost 200 different small plates are created to tempt your palate. Festival of the Holidays and Festival of the Arts are the smallest, with around 30-35 dishes each. Flower & Garden has over 45 dishes. The true food paradise is Food & Wine Festival, with 95 different dishes at the marketplaces. Food & Wine also has special food events around Epcot, at Disney resorts, and at Disney Springs, where chefs from around the world can play with ways to amuse your bouche. Add those to the marketplaces and there are well over 150 ways to magically munch during Food & Wine.

Who develops all these delicious dishes and makes sure they meet the high Disney culinary standards? It's often the chefs from your favorite World Showcase restaurants. "The chefs in each country decide on the dishes at the festival locations. We come up with ideas. Then we create and test and taste. And then refine and then taste again," explains Chef Bruno, the head chef at Les Chefs de France. "Then we share with the other chefs. All the dishes are also made in the kitchens in the countries. We have a huge kitchen in the France Pavilion where we make all the dishes served at the festival kiosks in France. The food is made in the kitchens and then plated at the kiosks."

How do you keep track of these tasty bites while at the festivals? With a passport book! For each festival, Epcot offers passport-size books that list each of the food kiosks, a checklist of the dishes and drinks, and a new addition, sheets of stickers. In the past, each kiosk would have a stamp and guests could ask the cast member to stamp their passport. This became a hassle for busy cast members and the stamps were sometimes misplaced. Now each book has a sheet of stickers and a space for you to mark the kiosks you have conquered. At the end of a successful festival journey you have a colorful memento of your gluttony. And who doesn't love stickers?

Epcot International Festival of the Arts

Festival of the Arts runs from January through mid-February and is the newest of the Epcot festivals, having debuted in 2017 on a Monday-Friday schedule. It brings the magic of the visual, culinary, and performing arts to Disney World. It returns in 2018, and will be open 7 days a week.

At Festival of the Arts you can step inside famous paintings, take classes from artistic masters, see Broadway-caliber productions, and indulge at the gourmet Food Studios. There are 10 different galleries featuring art from Disney greats Mary Blair and Herb Ryman. Make sure to visit the photo backdrops where you can hang in a boat with George Washington or become the Mona Lisa. According to cast member Nick, "This is a festival that combines food and art. Food is an art form in and of itself and it is on display at this Festival."

The food kiosks at Festival of the Arts are called Food Studios. In 2017, there were 8 Food Studios, from E=AT^2 featuring modernist cuisine (formerly called molecular gastronomy) to Cuisine Classique featuring new twists on classic dishes like ratatouille and chocolate chip cookies. "The coolest thing is the food," says Nick. "They make the most beautiful food and make it look like art. It's food that you sometimes don't want to eat because it's so pretty. But you do because it's so delicious."

Tips for enjoying Festival of the Arts:

 Make time to explore, as there is art to discover in nooks and crannies all around the park.

- Check out the festival merchandise. There are big-name artists like Thomas Kinkade and also local artisans at the event. There was even a person hand-painting shoes with Disney designs.
- Don't miss the giant paint-by-number. Each person is given paint and a square to fill. At the end of the festival there is this huge mural that thousands of people helped create. "It's like a giant community art project and you feel a sense of pride for having been a part of it," says Nick.
- Festival of the Arts is home to the Disney on Broadway Concert Series. The series featured live performances by Broadway stars singing songs from Disney classics like *Beauty and the Beast*, *Tarzan*, *Aladdin*, *Lion King*, and *The Little Mermaid*."

Epcot International Flower and Garden Festival

Flower & Garden usually runs from the beginning of March through the end of May. This festival is our favorite, as in addition to the food, Epcot comes alive with flowers and plants of every shape, size, and color.

Flower & Garden will hit all of your senses with gorgeous flower displays, interactive gardens and exhibits, fragrant blooms in gardens like Edible Flowers and Extraordinary Orchids, the Garden Rocks Concert Series, and the fresh tastes at the Outdoor Kitchens. Make sure you visit Butterflies on the Go and visit Inside the Gardenscape, a beautiful 3-D experience.

The food kiosks at Flower and Garden are called Outdoor Kitchens. Just the name sounds healthy. The food is focused on fresh, farm-to-table-style small plates and cocktails. Watermelon salad, the Urban Fairy Cocktail, and the Violet Lemonade, made famous by its deep purple color (and Instagram), are but a few of the treats found here.

Tips for enjoying the Flower & Garden Festival:

- Stop and smell the roses. Literally. Flower & Garden Festival is a time to slow down and pay attention to the details. Everywhere you look at Epcot there are topiaries of favorite Disney characters, gardens exploding with colors, and fragrant flowers and herbs. There's even an Epcot Egg-stravaganza Easter Egg Hunt.

- Look in all directions at Flower & Garden as you never know where you will see a gorgeous topiary or flower detail. In the UK Pavilion check out the roof of the main shop to find Peter Pan. In the model train area in World Showcase, look closely and you will see the Flower & Garden signage on the train station, colorful window boxes with tiny flowers, and potted plants in the town square.
- A good portion of the festival takes place in spring, which can be warm but not the fry-an- egg-on-the-sidewalk hot of Florida in June through August. In late May, it can get steamy. On hot days hit the Outdoor Kitchens early; most are open by 11am or a bit earlier. Or go later after it starts to cool off.
- Flower & Garden isn't just for gardeners, and if you're there with kids there are a number of ways to enjoy it. The best is the Play Gardens, small playgrounds dotted around the park. The Cars-themed playground near Test Track is a great location to take a rest while the kids play. Even at Disney World, a kid is a kid and a playground must be played at! Oliver enjoyed this playground as much as any of the rides at Epcot. While he played, Joe and I made trips to the different Outdoor Kitchens in the area and we had a nice picnic lunch in the park. There are also a number of kid-themed gardens. Kids of all ages enjoy the Egg-Stravaganza Easter Egg Hunt for the large Disney-character Easter eggs hidden around the pavilions.

Epcot International Food & Wine Festival

Food & Wine is the most popular Epcot festival. Every year Disney adds to it a few days or even a week. In 2017, it began at the end of August and ran a record 75 days to mid-November.

The Food & Wine Festival is all about the foods and drinks. There were 35 Marketplaces in 2017, the most of any festival, and over 20 more than at Flower & Garden. At Food & Wine, you can try over 200 different foods and drinks. Where else can you try so many different dishes prepared by 160 Disney chefs from 20 different countries in 1.25 miles?

What dishes? Everything. From beef skewers with boniato puree in Patagonia to fisherman's pie in Ireland to a Kung Fu Punch in China to Schinkennudeln in Germany. There are over 90 different small plates and over 100 ways to light your Disney buzz.

Tips for enjoying the Food & Wine Festival:

- Try the Tasting Sampler. This is a credential/voucher that gets you 8 different foods or drinks at the Food & Wine Marketplaces. You can purchase it at multiple locations around the festival. In 2017, the cost was $65, which included a limited-release Food & Wine trading pin. With the average price of a marketplace dish and cocktail being around $10-12, this can help add some money back into your Disney dining budget. You use your sampler as you walk around to the different marketplaces. There are some foods and drinks that may be excluded, but they'll be listed on the voucher. To get your money's worth, use the sampler for the most expensive items at the marketplaces, in particular cocktails.
- It can be pretty steamy in Florida during September and October. Standing in line and eating cheddar cheese soup when it's 95 degrees is not my idea of fun. To maximize your food and drink consumption, start early; most of the Marketplaces are open by 11am, some earlier. Then head to Future World to cool off for a few hours. Return to World Showcase around 4-5pm and finish the evening there.
- Food & Wine has become one of the most popular events at Disney not just for the food, but for the drinks as well. If drinking or being around folks who have been drinking is not your thing, avoid Epcot on Thursday through Sunday evenings during Food & Wine. During this time the World Showcase can feel more like a beer fest or pub crawl.
- If drinking in the park is your deal, and you want to leave the kids at home or with Disney babysitting so you can have a night of grown-up fun, this is an awesome time of year to do it. There are official tasting parties and concerts

and even unofficial Epcot pub crawls. You can add your drinks to the 360,000 beers or 300,000 wine servings dispensed during this event.

- Disney realizes that Food & Wine is probably not high on the list for most kids, but there are a few activities they might enjoy, such as Ratatouille Hide & Squeak, a scavenger hunt to find all the Remys hidden at each marketplace. Progress is tracked with stickers on a map. There is a cost, which basically pays for the Remy-food-themed pin you receive once all the Remys are found.
- Another kid-friendly activity is Agent P's World Showcase Adventure, an interactive game that will have you and your family going deep into the pavilions of World Showcase to solve various missions. The Agent P Adventure starts at a kiosk where friendly cast members dressed in the signature Agent P orange and teal give you a FONE (Field Operative Notification Equipment). We did the Adventure in 2015 during Food & Wine with Oliver. The FONE, a cell-phone-like device, gave Oliver instructions for different missions and showed funny clips from the show *Phineas & Ferb*. The missions will have you dashing around World Showcase, triggering special effects that have been sprinkled throughout the pavilions. It's similar to a scavenger hunt, but you are hunting for Dr. Doofenshmirtz, the goofy bad guy from the show.
- Agent P's World Showcase Adventure can definitely get a crowd's attention. There was a lot of giggling in Germany when Oliver activated the glockenspiel smack dab in the middle of the super-busy square. About 40 tired, sweaty guests were treated to a noisy Doofenshmirtz being chased by an angry blonde German woman with a giant club. In Japan, Oliver made Agent P speed by a crowd on a boat. A fellow guest asked, "Did that little boy do that? Can you do that again?" Definitely a magical Disney moment when a fellow guest asks your child to make the magic happen!

Epcot International Festival of the Holidays

Festival of the Holidays starts at the tail end of the Food & Wine Festival and runs until the end of the year—approximately mid- to late November through December 30. This festival is growing every year and the biggest change is the number of food offerings at the aptly named Holiday Kitchens.

Festival of the Holidays has so much to see. Each pavilion is decorated for the season and features holiday traditions. Many of the countries have storytellers sharing holiday stories and customs, like Pere Noel (France), La Befana (Italy), and even Mr. & Mrs. Claus at American Adventure. There are displays, the History of the Christmas Tree being one of my favorites. The highlight for many is the Candlelight Processional with celebrity narrators telling the Christmas story. This is a beautiful event with an orchestra, the Voices of Liberty, and a cast member choir as a singing Christmas tree.

The Holiday Kitchens offer traditional holiday dishes and drinks from around the world. Desserts are a big feature in many countries, so sample the stollen, a holiday fruitcake in Germany; panettone, an Italian Christmas cake in Italy; and cinnamon mochi cake in Japan. Holiday-themed cocktails are abundant, with traditional Christmas toddy in the UK and both grown-up and kid-friendly eggnog in American Adventure.

Tips for enjoying Festival of the Holidays:

- Grab a Festival of the Holidays passport so you can track the jolly treats you sample and the entertainment you enjoy. Check out the displays between countries, like the History of the Christmas Tree and the winter wonderland model train set.
- Osborne Spectacle of Lights has left Hollywood Studios, but you can still get a holiday decorations fix by walking the World Showcase.
- After the Candlelight Processional, there is a holiday-themed Illuminations, Epcot's firework show. Make sure to dress for Orlando in December. Yes, it is Orlando, but it's also December. Epcot can get chilly at

night around the lagoon, and shorts and t-shirts this time of year will often not keep you warm. You don't need a down puffy jacket, but a sweatshirt and pair of jeans will stop the shivers.

- Check out Spaceship Earth as you are leaving the park. Disney will wish you a good night in the different languages of the 11 World Showcase pavilions. With the smaller Christmas trees near the stage at Fountain View Plaza in the foreground and "Gute Nacht" in huge letters on Spaceship Earth in the background, it's a beautiful festive picture that puts you into the holiday spirit.

Epcot Festivals Tips

- One of the challenges of any Epcot festival is the lack of seating. A cheese plate from Ireland or a taco from Mexico are on-the-go friendly, but trying to eat short ribs with a knife and fork balanced on your kid's head takes away from the experience a bit. We did find a few hidden seating gems that can make eating more enjoyable. Joe, Oliver, and I enjoyed tacos on the steps of the Mexico pavilion and pastries on the ledge around the fountain in France, which has the added benefit of being a bit cooler because of the water. The benches by the buildings in China offer shade, comfort, and a scenic view, and the crates outside of the African outpost are a welcome respite when you're in the long stretch between countries. Or you can just stand in a circle taking bites and passing around whatever delectable treasure you've found.
- Go once the sun has gone down and it's cooler. Joe and I love food. We travel for food. We planned our last three vacations based on the fact that they were cities known for great food. During our trip to Food & Wine in 2015, there was so much to be excited about during the trip that I didn't realize until I was home how many more dishes I wish I had been able to try. My passport has far fewer checkmarks than I had been planning for. And when it's hot you just eat less. Had our feet not been ready to fall off and the 1/3 mile walk back to our room at Kidani

Village looming ahead, I may have been able to make another tasty trip around the World Showcase. When it was cooler, a lamb meatball with spicy tomato chutney would have hit the spot.

- Prioritize your food. I would have liked to try every single one of the dishes and cocktails on offer at Food & Wine. There were over 30 different cocktails, and even more wines, beers, and liquors like sake and vodka. Prior to the trip, I had made a list of what I wanted to try and it was so long I had to prioritize, making an "A" and a "B" list. On my list were 31 dishes or cocktails our group needed to try. We spent from 9:15am to almost 7pm at Epcot, primarily in World Showcase, and I tried 12 of the 31 dishes/cocktails on my list.
- On a tight dining budget? Purchase a festival gift card at any store carrying festival merchandise or at the Festival Center, typically located near Mission: SPACE. Put your daily budget on the card and when you're out, you're out. The cashiers at each food kiosk can tell you how much remains, and it makes a great festival souvenir.

Urban Fairy Cocktail

You'll find the Urban Fairy Cocktail at Epcot's Flower & Garden Festival (in 2017, it was served at the Urban Farm Eats kitchen). Served cold, it comes in a festival-friendly plastic martini glass with a slice of fresh cucumber, and is quite potent. The different liquors are not specified, but it definitely includes absinthe. The cocktail has a bitter, anise, black licorice flavor, softened only slightly by the icy cold temperature.

I don't know for sure, but I think this cocktail got its name because of the absinthe, which is also called the Green Fairy. Absinthe is sometimes called the Green Fairy because of its bright green color and reputation for causing hallucinations, which has not been scientifically proven. But, in my experience, if you drink enough of any potent liquor, it can result in thinking you are seeing double, or fairies.

Ordering Tip: Have this cocktail with a friend and plan to drink it quickly. It really is a sipping cocktail, but tastes better cold.

The Flower & Garden Festival is home to many refreshing, bright cocktails with ingredients like edible flowers and cucumber. Just like the food, the cocktails have a fresh, healthy vibe.

V

Victoria & Albert's Villain Cupcake

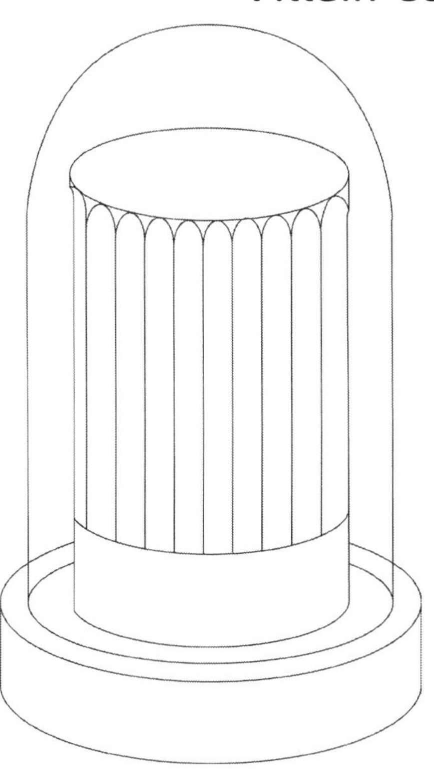

Victoria & Albert's

Victoria & Albert's, the most luxurious and distinctive culinary experience in Orlando, is in the Grand Floridian Resort and Spa. It has received the most accolades of any Disney restaurant. The artistic plating, fresh ingredients, impeccable service, and elegant dishes make it the restaurant of choice for special occasions. It is on the bucket list of foodies around the world.

Victoria & Albert's is called the ultimate in fine dining and is unlike any other restaurant at Disney World. Don't expect to see chicken fingers, strollers or fanny packs. But, here are a few things you can expect:

- A few days before your dinner, the restaurant will contact you asking about food allergies, requests, or any specific foods you do not like. For example, if you'll be at Victoria & Albert's during asparagus season, expect to see a lot of asparagus in the meal. If you don't like asparagus, the phone call is the perfect time to mention it. Allergic to peanuts? No worries, they are very accommodating, just make sure to tell them sooner rather than later.
- There is a strict dress code. Flip-flops and Mickey ears need to stay in your room. However, this is the perfect place to show off that new Disney Dooney & Burke bag. There is a stool for your purse.
- The restaurant has only 18 tables. The ultimate culinary experience is the Chef's Table. This table is in the kitchen and you and your party will be served special treats from the chef and his team. And you can bug him with questions throughout the meal.
- Don't plan to see fireworks afterward. The meal will last about 4 hours and you may be so full you will want to be carried back to your room.
- Be prepared to spend at least $1,000 for a meal for two. Your server will also offer a few different upgrades, perhaps an additional Kobe beef course or the wine pairing.
- If you want to do a wine pairing, share it. The wine pours are generous. By about the sixth course you will

be feeling the effects of six half glasses of wine and won't even remember or have the room for the cheese course or multiple dessert courses. Watch your drink consumption in general. Four hours is a long time to be sipping on wine or cocktails, for the belly and the brain!

- This is not the restaurant for a picky eater. Victoria & Albert's features a prix fixe menu, with either 8 or 10 small courses of the chef's choosing.
- Like most things Disney, Victoria & Albert's is a marathon, not a sprint. Making it through as many as 10 courses may not seem too difficult. The plates aren't that big, right? Wrong! There are 8-10 dishes in addition to the amuse bouche, bread, wine, and any other bites the chef decides to send your way.
- Over the course of this four-hour meal, the chef will take your taste buds on a magical journey of every taste imaginable: sweet, savory, rich, umami. The culinary influences may be French in one plate, Asian the next, and then a play on American comfort food. Each plate will look like art and will have the freshest ingredients and painstaking attention to detail.
- The first course is an amuse bouche. This is a small dish, typically one or two bites, that is intended to wake up your palate. Typically it is a light dish that explodes with fresh flavors.
- Different breads come between each course. Each bread has its own butter. Pace yourself. It may be tasty, but you will quickly regret eating all those carbs.
- Your server will notice and may ask if you don't clear your plate. This has happened to me at a few high-end dinners and it can be a bit mortifying. Prevent this by asking to have the pacing slowed down a bit so there is more time between courses. Also make sure you let them know of any items you really dislike or are allergic to. Be careful with this list. If you really only like chicken nuggets and pizza, and you hate the idea of anything green or from the sea, save yourself the $1,000 and try a different restaurant.

 At the end of the meal, when the last thing you want to see is more food, out comes a dessert cart full of decadent take-home sweet treats. They are perfect to pull out the next day when you've digested and the wine has worn off.

Most important: relax, enjoy yourself, and know you belong there. Quite a few Victoria & Albert's diners have shared that they felt horribly out of place and were just waiting for the waiter to call them on it. Don't get wasted and dance on the table. If you walk in wearing a swimsuit and fanny pack, they will say something. But this is a fine dining restaurant with highly trained professionals who want each and every guest to have a magical experience. They want you to enjoy the harpist playing Disney covers. They love that you are so excited that there is a stool just for your purse. They feel pride when you are amazed what the chef can do with duck. They will even happily do a photo with you at the end of the meal. Just make sure to use your table manners, don't drink too much, and savor the magic.

Villain Cupcake

The villain cupcake is served at the Happily Ever After Fireworks Dessert Party at Magic Kingdom. This event is all about desserts. If dessert is not your thing, and you prefer fries over chocolate cake, it's not for you.

Event Tip: Eat dinner before you come. The only source of real food at this event is cheese, crackers, and fruit in the kids kabobs. Also, make sure to scope out the entire dessert scene before making your selection. There were 14 different dessert options during our 2017 party. If you prefer to have your cupcake followed by a glug of Diet Coke, buy a soda before coming to the party. Sodas were not part of the drink selection at our party and it's not clear if they will be added any time soon.

There are two main locations for the desserts: a buffet style that is on the terrace and the kids section, which we found had the tastiest options. The drinks are near the kids section and include coffee, water, lemonade, milk, and sparkling cider. The sparkling cider is pretty sweet, but serving it in champagne flutes makes it feel fancy. The dessert offerings are constantly changing. During the party we attended in May 2017 they included:

- Red velvet and villain cupcakes.
- Gigantic chocolate-covered strawberries with dark and white chocolate, a strawberry tart, and pineapple delight. We overheard a guest say it reminded them of Dole Whip.
- Many different types of macarons, including pistachio, lemon, raspberry, vanilla, coffee, and chocolate. Our favorite was the pistachio; the nuttiness kept it from being too sweet. The coffee macaron had a nice bitterness to it. Put three macarons on a plate to make your own hidden Mickey.
- A chocolate almond cake with a plump raspberry on top, cheesecake brownie bites, and a chocolate marshmallow tart with two pieces of crispy dark chocolate on the top.
- For the kids, there were kids kabobs, a "decorate your own cupcake or cookie" station, and a "make your own ice cream" station.
- No dessert party is complete without a Mickey treat. The Oreo Mickey Treat was a chocolate tart base with a pile of frosting topped by two mini chocolate cookies, made to look like Mickey ears.

We were a bit disappointed with the quality of the desserts for the price of the event. We were really paying for the ability to avoid standing in the Main Street crowd during Happily Ever After as we both hate crowds and there is no longer a FastPass+ to sit on the hub grass for the show. The cost was about $120 for the two of us and we ate 2 or 3 desserts apiece. The kids kabobs were the highlight for me, with a plump strawberry, marshmallow, rice Krispy treat, pineapple, and brownie that you slide onto a red Mickey straw and then dip in chocolate sauce.

The villain cupcake was a dark chocolate cake, topped with a generous helping of deep purple frosting and dark chocolate round crunchies on top. It looked villainous and was very photogenic, being the perfect shade of purple for pics with my first book, *The Not-So-Evil Stepmother in the Most Magical Place on Earth*.

Purple is just a villain color, right? The cupcake looked far more delectable than it was. The purple frosting tasted of the dye that made it purple and the chocolate cake was too sweet. The combination of the very bitter frosting with an overly sweet cake was not good. Most of the desserts tasted factory-made. Having had the delicious Grey Stuff at Be Our Guest and many tasty treats from Main Street Confectionery, both of which were a 5-minute walk away from this event, the lack of quality desserts in relation to the cost of the event was disappointing. We were basically paying for a pleasant place to watch the night show. It was worth the cost to avoid the crowds.

W

Waffle, Mickey Shaped

The Wave

Wedding Cake

Whispering Canyon Café

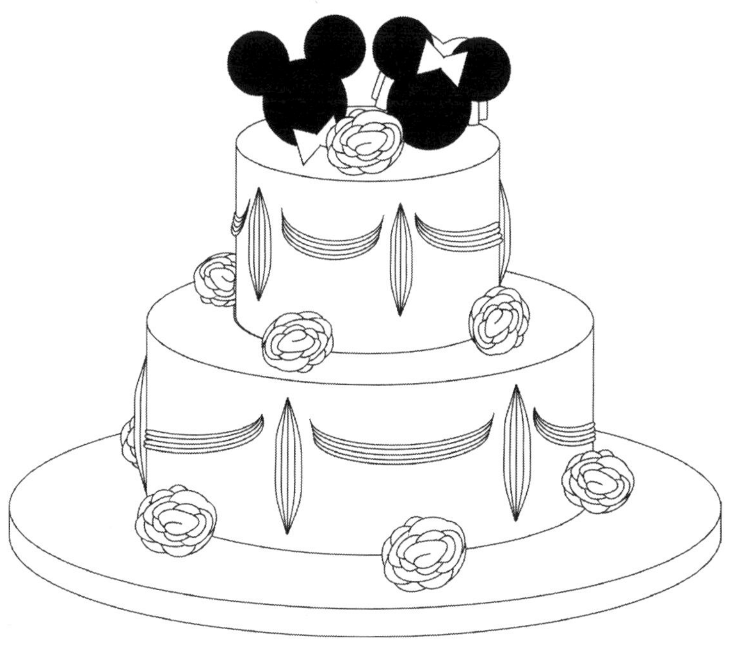

Waffle, Mickey Shaped

Around 1,700 Mickey waffles are served each day at Chef Mickey's alone. Over 20 other Disney World restaurants serve them as well.

Mickey waffles are a Disney staple and available year round at breakfast. You can munch on a Mickey waffle while strolling down Main Street, by the pool at Siesta Cantina at Coronado Springs, or while hanging with Mickey at Chef Mickey's. That might be weird, though. Eating a waffle shaped like his head in front of Mickey...

These little Mickey-shaped nuggets of goodness are a must for any Disney trip. If you hit a breakfast buffet at just the right time, you can get one piping hot from the waffle iron. It will be crispy on the outside and moist on the inside. Add a dollop of fluffy whipped cream with crunchy bacon, that just happens to get a bit of maple syrup on it, and it's the perfect sweet/savory breakfast.

Location Tip: Mickey waffles are available at breakfast (until 11am) at Plaza Ice Cream Parlor in Magic Kingdom. They come topped with powdered sugar, strawberries, and a side of bacon. Who knew? If I had known it was this easy to get a Mickey waffle fix, Plaza Ice Cream would have been my next stop on Main Street after a must-have Starbucks.

Cast member Nick has worked at Disney for over two years and grew up in central Florida, so he has eaten a lot of Mickey waffles in his day. One of his most memorable Mickey waffle moments happened during breakfast at 'Ohana in the Polynesian Village:

> Our friends ran the Princess 5K and afterwards they needed to carb load, so we had breakfast at 'Ohana at Polynesian. They bring you out one of those huge metal serving trays caterers use. It is chock full of sausage, hash browns, eggs, and a few pounds of Mickey waffles. You dig in and eat until you're ready to explode. Then

> your waiter sees that you're running low and brings you another one! Even I still get excited about having Mickey waffles, but 7 pounds of them later I never wanted to see a Mickey waffle again. When Mickey waffles come in a trough of breakfast food it truly is the ultimate Mickey waffle experience.

Concerned about having Mickey waffle withdrawal? No worries. There are Mickey Waffle irons for sale.

If you're like Nick and have had your fill of eating Mickey waffles, or you're gluten- or carb-free, you can wear your waffles on a t-shirt. Or on Mickey ears. Your favorite pooch can even get in on the waffle action with a Mickey waffle dog toy. But the ultimate non-edible Mickey waffle is a Vinlymation. It has a Mickey waffle head with a body that looks as if it's made of syrup with more syrup dripping down the ears and neck. It is one of the only Mickey waffles that is diet friendly.

The Wave

The Wave...of American Flavors at the Contemporary Resort serves American cuisine, but not of the "diner" variety. Instead of burgers and fries, it has dishes like short ribs with goat cheese polenta.

Make sure to try the bacon and eggs appetizer with rich, salty pork belly and a perfectly cooked egg with creamy smoked cheddar grits. Like many restaurants, The Wave has a pricey light-up cup to hold your child's beverage.

The Wave also has a lounge area where grown-ups can escape from the magic. Disney doesn't prohibit kids from coming into this area, but in our time there, no kids ventured in. True to its oceanic name, The Wave features an abundance of blue lighting and wave-like patterns on the walls and furnishings with a contemporary vibe.

The lounge has a bar area with the typical TV screens showing multiple sports, so Joe and I chose to check out a seating area just off the bar that was aglow in the bright blue signature lights. My cocktail was blue and blended right in with the decor.

With recent additions in 2016 and 2017 like Nomad Lounge, Tiffins, and Art Smith's Homecomin' at Disney Springs, Disney has been upping its cocktail game. Cocktails at these locations feature fresh fruits and herbs and taste less syrupy sweet.

The cocktails at The Wave were okay, but a bit on the flashy, looking-cool-over-taste side. The people-watching at the lounge was interesting, to say the least. There was a raucous group of couples that were downing shots with their cocktails, and a giggling group of women in their 20s that we suspected were part of a bachelorette party.

Location Tip: The Wave Lounge has a small food menu featuring a cheese board, burger, and a salad. If you're in a hurry and don't have a reservation for the restaurant, sit at the bar to grab a quick bite.

Ordering Tip: For breakfast, you can order from the menu or partake of The Wave's breakfast-only buffet.

Wedding Cake

Disney wedding cakes come in a variety of flavors and fillings. Depending on the location of the wedding, over 200 different cakes are available based on flavor and filling combinations. The Grand Floridian bakery does the wedding cakes for its Wedding Pavilion as well as for most weddings on Disney World property.

In 2005, we had a Disney wedding at the gazebo between Yacht and Beach Club. When doing one of the smaller fairytale wedding ceremonies, now called the Escape, a champagne and cake celebration is part of the package. For our wedding, the entire ceremony and celebration set-up was done before we arrived. This meant that the cake was at the wedding and taunting us, especially the kids, for the entire ceremony.

After the ceremony, we had a Fairytale Cuvee champagne toast. We upgraded and also added a bottle of sparkling apple cider, which went over like gangbusters with Nate, Maggie,

Annie, and Austin. We have a great photo of the four of them toasting Joe and me. They all had fun pretending they were drinking actual champagne.

Our cake looked enchanting. We had stayed very basic and just had a yellow cake with a buttercream-frosting filling. It was three tiers piled high with white frosting that looked like clouds with Groom Mickey and Bride Minnie perched on top. There are even flavor combinations like chocolate cake with amaretto mousse with almond crunch or lemon cake with raspberry mousse and fresh raspberries available, so wedding cakes at Disney taste as magical as they look.

If you've always wondered what it's like to have a Disney Fairytale Wedding, check out my first book, *The Not-So-Evil Stepmother in the Most Magical Place on Earth*.

Whispering Canyon Café

Whispering Canyon Café is in the lobby of Wilderness Lodge, and you'll hear it before you see it: there is a lot of whooping, hollering, and smells of barbecue chicken.

The food is "Old West" style. The café is open for breakfast, lunch, and dinner. Breakfast is a standard menu with eggs, oatmeal, and Chad's Chocolate Chip Buttermilk Flapjacks. Lunch is all about sandwiches and burgers. Dinner has western favorites for entrees and upscale western appetizers including a pulled pork spring roll and chilled yellow tomato soup. The most popular entrée is the all-you-care-to-enjoy skillet with ribs, pork, chicken, beef, sausage, and a wide selection of ranch favorites on the side like cowboy-style baked beans and mashed Yukon potatoes.

Ordering Tip: If meat is not your thing, Whispering Canyon also has salmon and a crispy rainbow trout.

Try the fresh-baked cornbread and a moonshine cocktail. There are a number of moonshine offerings on the menu.

Whispering Canyon Café is a sprawling place. If you don't mind the noise and want to be part of the action, ask if you can be in the main dining room. Behind the dining room, to the side of the kitchen, is a space with a few smaller tables near a fireplace. Beyond that are a few tables that run along the back of the restaurant and are situated in an area that resembles the front porch of a country house.

In 2015, we went to Whispering Canyon to celebrate Oliver's 5th birthday. After playing Legos with Dad in the waiting area, we were seated. A petite, friendly woman came over and introduced herself as our waitress Lazy Susan. Upon hearing it was the day before Oliver's 5th birthday and seeing the birthday button, she started showing the surprisingly loud voice contained in her small frame. We ordered up a family meal with BBQ meats, baked beans, corn bread, and potatoes. Oliver went for a grilled cheese.

The food at Whispering Canyon is good, but it's really about the meal activities and entertaining cast members. During our short dinner, Joe and about 20 other dads sang and did the "I'm a Little Teapot" dance. Oliver had a race around the dining room with a fake horse on a stick and Lazy Susan yelled at Oliver about eating his dinner multiple times.

Ordering Tip: Ask for ketchup.

For Oliver's birthday moment, Lazy Susan demanded all the folks in our section, including this cute young couple who were unsuccessfully trying to have a romantic dinner, sing "Happy Birthday." Later, when this couple asked Susan to take a picture of them in front of the fireplace, she invited Oliver into the photo. Oliver described it best: "Susan yelled my name during dinner and then had me get a picture with these people I didn't know. They even sang "Happy Birthday" to me. Susan made me laugh, but she was crazy!"

Location Tip: Whispering Canyon is one of the best places at Disney World to celebrate birthdays. If you're shy, be ready to be embarrassed as the servers make a lot of racket about birthdays and make absolute strangers sing to you. There are cupcakes involved, so it may be worth a minute of humiliation.

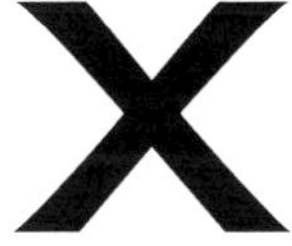

Xtra-Large Margarita Flight

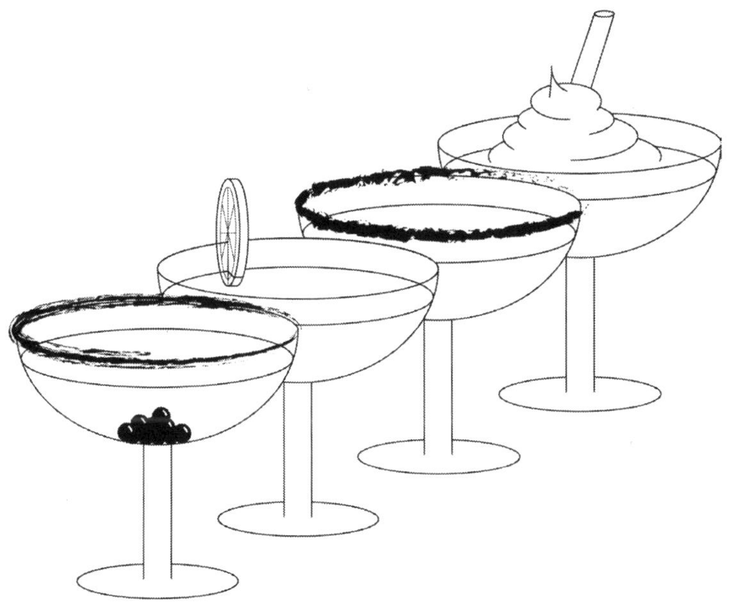

Xtra-Large Margarita Flight

When they run out of the shot glasses for the margarita flight at Rix Lounge at Coronado Springs, they serve it "xtra-large style." A typical size margarita flight is available most of the time.

After a long day of Magic Kingdom, cheerleading rehearsal, and eating dinner after 10pm, all I needed during my trip in 2016 was a little something to help my mind and shoulders relax and help calm my head so I could sleep. At Disney World, I really do get too excited to sleep!

Austin's cheer rehearsal ended around 10:30pm, so a few hundred hungry teenagers descended on the poor chefs at Pepper Market. Even with seating for 400, Pepper Market was packed. Rather than deal with the wall of sound that is teenage girls, I went across the way to the quiet, comfortable Rix Lounge.

Location Tip: Typically, lounges are for 21 and older. The manager said the Lounge was 21 and over only. However, Pepper Market had run out of seating and the manager gave up after the 50th parent walked in with their kid and said, "I'm eating here." On a typical day, if you have kids with you, order your food to go and pop over to Pepper Market seating or outside to the seating along the lakefront.

Rix Lounge is home to the delicious and filling chips and dip. The chips are house-made and very crunchy. They're lightly dusted with a BBQ powder, avoiding the grittiness of typical BBQ chips. The dip is a caramelized French onion. Each bite is bursting with flavor and a mix of textures from the combination of crispy, salty chips and creamy dip with chunks of sweet, perfectly caramelized onion.

Ordering tip: Rix Lounge, like many Disney restaurants, has generous portion sizes. The chips and dip could have easily served three with some leftovers.

The menu featured any number of effective-looking cocktails, but I decided to be a bit adventurous and try the margarita flight. It included five different margaritas that are typically served in small shot glasses. Five shot glasses of potent margarita is enough for a lightweight like myself, so imagine my surprise when the friendly bartender started to bring over plastic tumblers 2/3 full of brightly colored liquids. “We ran out of the shot glasses,” he said with a devilish grin. “Enjoy.”

The flavors included:

- **Mango Blueberry Basil.** A soft orange color with a bright orange spicy salt on the rim. This was one of the sweetest of the group. I would have liked to taste more of the basil.
- **Classic.** A pale yellow with a clear salty rim. The classic is a good, solid margarita, but flavor wise felt a bit boring next to the others.
- **Blood Orange.** A bright pink drink with a pink rim that was a bit too spicy for my tastes. The margarita itself was the perfect blend of sweet and tangy.
- **Pineapple.** Orangey yellow with a pink rim that was like eating a pineapple Dum-Dum. Not being a big fan of Pineapple, this was my least favorite.
- **Jalapeno.** Bright yellow with a sweet pink rim, the gentle heat from the jalapeno balanced the sugar in the rim and the natural sweetness from the lime. The drink hits your tongue nice and cool, but then you get the warmth as the jalapeno kicks in.

The five together made a beautiful rainbow of potent margarita goodness. It would have been so much more fun if I’d had someone to share it with, but it was only the teens around. Of the five, the jalapeno was the favorite, followed by the blood orange, classic, mango blueberry basil, and last the pineapple. The spicy jalapeno paired nicely with my chips and dip and was the only one I finished. After multiple tasting sips of each, and finishing the Jalapeno, locating my room in the Casitas building was interesting.

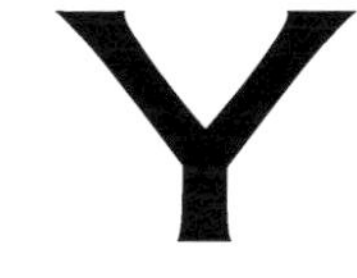

Yak & Yeti Yogurt Parfait

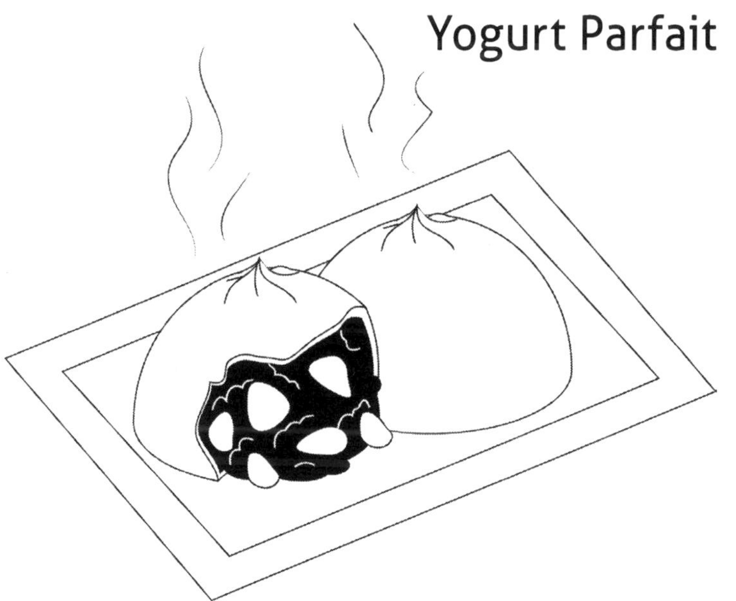

Yak & Yeti

Yak & Yeti is located in Asia at Animal Kingdom. As you approach it from Africa, you feel a distinctive shift in the decorations and style as the buildings become more colorful. Expedition Everest peeks over the treetops in the distance.

The restaurant serves traditional Asian cuisine. The building is a beautiful purple color with ornate windows and a subtle sign. Inside there is dark carved furniture, beautiful artwork, Asian sculptures, and colorful Tibetan prayer flags scattered about.

Location Tip: Yak & Yeti is two stories with a gorgeous teak wood staircase leading to a bright blue second floor. If people watching is your thing, ask to sit on the second floor near the windows.

Make sure to try the dim sum basket with extra pork siu mai. The siu mai are BBQ pork buns steamed on banana leaves. These little buns are bursting with flavor. The inside is sweet barbecued pork that is surrounded by a soft white bun, almost like really tasty Wonder bread. As the buns are steamed, the bread gets soft and flavored by the meaty pork and tangy barbecue sauce.

Yogurt Parfait

The yogurt parfait, available at most resort quick-service locations, including Pepper Market at Coronado Springs, is the product of a build-your-own yogurt bar with a variety of yogurt flavors, fresh fruit, and granola toppings. Go traditional with a vanilla yogurt with strawberry layers, topped with a bit of granola. Or get the pre-made version with honey yogurt, fresh fruit, and your choice of toppings.

Every morning, my mom would build her own parfait at Pepper Market at Coronado Springs and then put it in the fridge for a healthy late-night snack. Both of my parents found the breakfast options at Pepper Market generous and reasonably priced.

Location Tip: At Coronado Springs, grab your food to go and head out the door toward the lake to enjoy the seating right at the water's edge. If you're there during the cooler months, you may even catch a cast member drawing your favorite Disney character on the sidewalk.

Z

Zimbabwean Soda

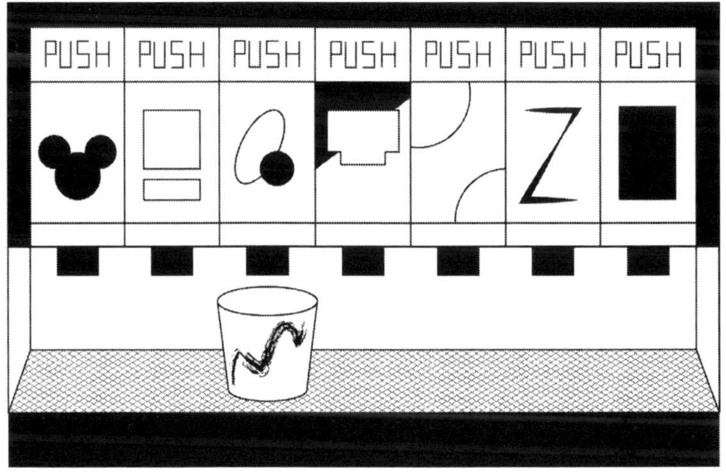

Zimbabwean Soda

Ever wondered what a soda from Zimbabwe tastes like? Or what Coca-Cola flavor is popular in Japan? At Club Cool, the Coca-Cola sampling center in Epcot, you can find out.

Club Cool is not to be missed. It's tucked away near Innoventions West, just before you get to The Land Pavilion. During our 2005 trip it was very quiet and felt like a hidden gem. During our visit in 2015 we discovered that was no longer true. The place was packed.

At Club Cool you can sample different sodas from different countries. It is a large, brightly lit room that looks like a Coca-Cola merchandise truck burst in it. There are a number of tasting stations, featuring the eight different flavors. Next to each machine are little Dixie cups. And it's free!

The flavors do change and are proof that taste buds can vary as you go around the world. There are typically eight different flavors. We recommend giving all of them at least a small sip. In 2015 we tried:

- Inca Kola (Peru) is like drinking fizzy bubblegum. Everyone likes gum.
- Guarana Kuat (Brazil) was a popular drink during the Olympics and tastes of apples and berries.
- Sparletta (Zimbabwe) is a raspberry-cream soda that I found very sweet. Raspberry is a subtle fruit and it only shows through a bit in this drink. It has a whole lot of cream, not too much raspberry.
- VegiBeta (Japan) is a little odd. It's not carbonated and is fruit flavored with apricot and passion fruit. Not one of my favorites, but Joe likes it.
- Bibo (South Africa). This one is not carbonated. It can be a surprise when you're expecting fizz.
- Fanta Pineapple (Greece).
- Fanta Melon Frosty (Thailand) is melon flavored and one of my favorites.
- Beverly (Italy).

Like all things Disney, change happens. In 2013, Club Cool swapped most of the flavors for new ones. My favorite Smart Watermelon from China and the kid-favorite Lift Apple from Mexico were gone. Lesson learned. If you find a flavor you love, have a few cups. Or search for it at the restaurants in Animal Kingdom. Quite a few of the soda flavors have migrated from Epcot over to the Harambe Market. Pair the Sparberry from Zimbabwe or Bibo from South Africa with a curry sausage for an authentic African meal.

APPENDIX A

Dole Whip, Turkey Legs and More Ways to Taste the Magic

Just in case 35 foods and 36 restaurants isn't enough to fill your tasting list, here are a few additional ways to taste the magic from A-Z. Disney fans on Instagram shared these ideas for the Disney Eats from A-Z Food Challenge. Read all about that challenge in the next appendix.

- Baklava from @summerlovesdisney. Find it in Epcot at the Morocco food kiosk during most of the festivals or at Spice Road Table and Restaurant Marrakesh.
- Chocolate-covered pretzels from @adventures.with.carissa. Head to Main Street Confectionery in Magic Kingdom.
- Dole Whip from @rachiedawns. Dole Whip is being added to more menus. Find it in Aloha Isle at Magic Kingdom, Tamu Tamu in Africa at Animal Kingdom, Pineapple Lanai in the Polynesian Resort, and at a few Epcot festivals.
- Eggs in Purgatory, aka Two Eggs Poached Underwater @summerlovesdisney. Head to Trattoria at the Board-Walk Inn. This restaurant is also home to the new Bon Voyage character meal featuring Ariel and Prince Eric and Rapunzel and Finn.
- Falafel from @wishesdishes_wdwdelights. Falafel is one of those Disney foods that pops up and then goes away just as quickly. There is sometimes a stand called Mr. Kamal's at Animal Kingdom near the Yak & Yeti restaurant that is rumored to have the best falafel.

- Macarons from @summerlovesdisney. Head to Les Halles Boulangerie in the France Pavilion at Epcot.
- Pretzel in Germany from @_followthedisneymagic. Head to the Germany Pavilion in Epcot.
- Quiche from @main_st_brown. There are a few places to savor a quiche, including Le Halles Boulangerie-Patisserie in the France Pavilion at Epcot.
- The sweet-and-spicy chicken waffle sandwich from @crazyholley. This one comes and goes at Sleepy Hollow in Fantasyland at Magic Kingdom.
- Turkey legs from @crazyholley. With 1.6 million turkey legs consumed at Disney World each year, you can find them throughout the parks.
- Umngqusho from @summerlovesdisney. Have an adventure and this dish at Sanaa in Kidani Village at Animal Kingdom Lodge. It's on the dinner menu.
- Zebra Dome from @themainstreetmoms. They win the prize for having a suggestion for the toughest letter. Find it at Boma in the Animal Kingdom Lodge.

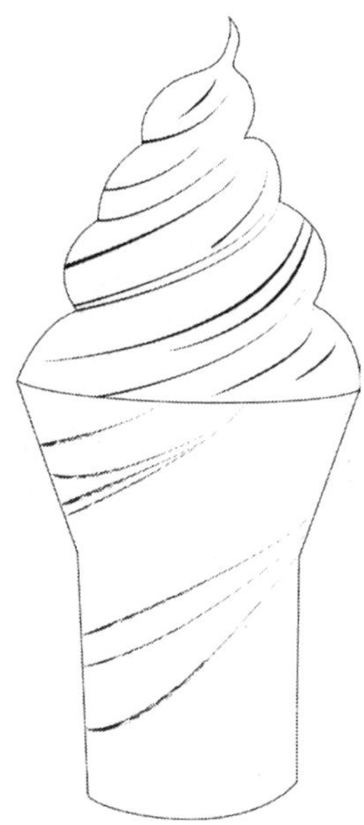

APPENDIX B

Disney Dining Challenge

Everyone loves a good challenge. And when that challenge involves food, it's even better. In 2016, I took on a Disney Eats from A-Z Challenge, answering the question: What does it take to eat the alphabet at Disney World? This challenge involved eating one dish for each letter of the alphabet in only 4 days (3 full days and 2 half-days). With 26 letters, that works out to about 7 eats per day.

I had help with the challenge in the form of my 16-year-old son Austin. In December 2016 Austin and I made the trek to Walt Disney World so he could be in the Varsity Spirit Spectacular, a cheerleading event held in Magic Kingdom, and so I could take my food challenge.

The holidays are a magical time at Walt Disney World: the decorations, special events, and my favorite thing, food.

Before we left I did some research and discovered that items starting with J, U, and Z would be particularly tricky. I was nervous that I was biting off more than I could chew... But if you're ever in a Disney bind, try social media. There are thousands of accounts on Instagram devoted to the Mouse. With some help from my new friends on Instagram, I had a plan.

This plan involved photos. Since I'm not really a fan of having my picture taken, I decided to use three adorable Disney Tsum Tsum stepmothers as proof of the amount of food consumed. These stepmoms included the Evil Queen from *Snow White*, Lady Tremaine from *Cinderella*, and a custom stepmother Tsum my daughter-in-law created of me. Yes, having a Tsum of yourself is as cool as it sounds.

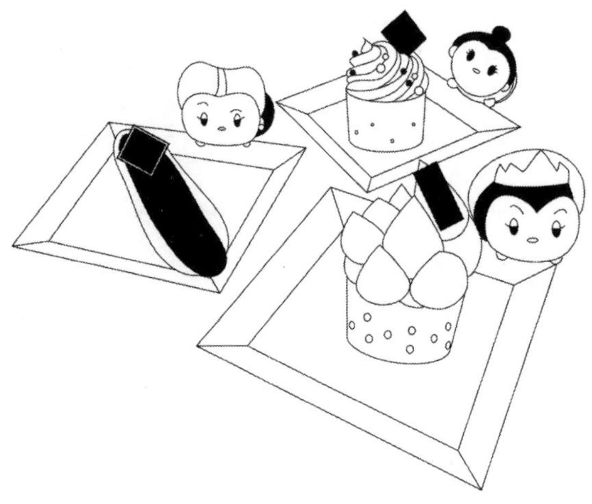

Day One: Wednesday

DISHES 1 AND 2. Empanadas and black beans from Pepper Market at Coronado Springs Resort. The black beans from Pepper Market were my favorite taste of the day and there were some good ones. Pepper Market is well known by Disney experts as a great place for a quick bite. The black beans have just the right amount of spicy kick and have just a touch of cilantro to add a pop of citrusy freshness. They are a mix of mashed and full beans so you get bursts of meatiness with a salty bite from the sprinkle of fresh queso on top.

DISH 3. Churros from Pepper Market, the first food stop on our trip. We had an early flight, arriving into Orlando just after 9am. After Magical Express, checking in, and finding our room, it was lunchtime and we were starving. This was my first time staying at Coronado Springs. The grounds are gorgeous, with fountains, colorful flowers, and the buildings are all brightly painted in peaches and teals. Like most Disney resorts, Coronado Springs is massive. We were fortunate to have a Casitas room, which is the closest to the lobby and the convention center.

DISH 4. Vanilla ice cream in the Ocean Beach Sea Salt Caramel Sundae at Ghirardelli Ice Cream Shop in Disney Springs.

Day 1 and B, C, E and V are done! Not quite the goal of seven, but this was a half-day so not a bad start. Lesson learned: balance the sweet with the salty. After only a few bites of the sundae, I was on a sugar high that kept me up well past midnight.

Day Two: Thursday

DISH 1. Frappuccino from Starbucks on Main Street in Magic Kingdom. Most of my mornings start with a Frappuccino and being at Disney World is no exception.

DISHES 2 AND 3. Icing on a Krispy treat from Main Street Confectionery in Magic Kingdom

DISHES 4, 5, AND 6. All at Be Our Guest in Magic Kingdom, starting with potato leek soup. Many French bistros feature a cold potato soup called vichyssoise. The potato leek soup at Be Our Guest is a take on this French staple, but is served warm. It features the same flavors of salty potato and leeks with a hefty serving of cream. The soup was rich and creamy with a little kick at the end. Along with the soup I had the roast beef sandwich and, for dessert, the Master's Cupcake.

DISHES 7 AND 8. Éclair a' l'orange and lemon meringue cupcake at Be Our Guest. The desserts here are not to be missed. My go-to is always the Master's Cupcake. The dessert menu does change a bit, but the Master's Cupcake is a staple we have seen every time. On this trip, we also tried the lemon meringue cupcake. This dessert looks like a plate of sunshine. It starts with a creamy vanilla sponge cake with a burst of citrus from the tangy lemon curd hiding inside. The cake is a beautiful happy yellow and is topped with piles of flamed fluffy-white meringue icing and a yellow-white chocolate square. If you are a lemon sweets lover, give this a try.

DISH 9. Watermelon raspberry smoothie at Café Rix in Coronado Springs. After all that food at Be Our Guest, dinner was the last thing on our minds. In addition to the appetizing

Pepper Market, Coronado Springs also has a quick-service venue called Café Rix which has a bakery section with delectable ways to make up all those calories burned by walking in the parks. It's also a great place for a smoothie. After poring over the menu and not finding the perfect smoothie option for my taste buds, a friendly cast member (Drew) offered to make me a custom smoothie. I just shared flavors I liked and he worked his magic. The end result was light with flavors of fresh watermelon and a slight tartness from the raspberry. It was also a beautiful soft pink color, like the ribbon detail on Rapunzel's dress.

DISH 10. XL Margarita flight at Rix Lounge in Coronado Springs.

Day 2 and F, I, L, K, M, O, R, W, X, and Y are done! Ten letters in one day makes up for the short list the day before. Having three different desserts at Be Our Guest is an effective way to get through many letters, and to make your pants fit a bit tighter the next morning. Ending the night with a flight of very large margaritas ensured insomnia was not a problem this evening.

Day Three: Friday

DISH 1. Dolce Cinnamon Coffee at Café Rix in Coronado Springs. Just like the custom smoothie from yesterday, the cast members at Café Rix did it again and made me a custom coffee. It was creamy and the cinnamon syrup gave it the taste of Christmas on the rocks.

DISH 2. Holiday Eats. Throughout Disney World there are tastes of the holidays. You can get special holiday cookies during Mickey's Very Merry Christmas Party at Magic Kingdom and there are a number of special festive pastries in all the parks. Epcot has the International Festival of the Holidays with holiday kitchens sprinkled around World Showcase. It was like a holiday-themed version of Food & Wine. Austin and I had a long list of jolly eats, but a few highlights were the Mickey gingerbread men, Mickey Santa Rice Krispies, beef tamales, and the holiday sandwich.

DISH 3. Avocado crema at Feast of the Three Kings Kitchen in Epcot. The avocado crema was atop the shredded beef tamale from the Three Kings kiosk. Often the festival servings are a few bites, but this tamale was surprisingly large. The shredded beef was tender and well seasoned with a variety of spices. The tamale shell was very thick, more like cornbread than the typical thin husky tamale shell. This was definitely a treat to eat at a table with a knife and fork. The highlight was the earthy light-green avocado crema that was flavorful and delicious. It was akin to a whipped guacamole. I could have definitely done with more.

DISH/DRINK 4. Jalapeno margarita at Epcot's San Angel Inn.

DISH 5. Queso fundido at San Angel Inn. This restaurant features up-scale Mexican food in one of the most unexpectedly beautiful dining locations at Epcot: the Mexico Pavilion. I ordered the queso fundido to fulfill the Q in the challenge, knowing my options would be limited. Good choice! Want to get your teenager to try something new? Take them to San Angel.

DISHES 6 AND 7. Tostada de Tinga and Zucchini on Tacos de Vegetales at San Angel Inn. San Angel Inn helped me check two very difficult letters off the list: Q and Z. There are a number of delectable and zesty entrees. Not being able to make a decision, two of my fellow diners and I decided to try a few different appetizers. Austin had the carne asada. This is a beautiful dish consisting of a perfectly cooked New York strip steak, with a cheese enchilada, beans, and red bell peppers. The rest of us shared the Tostadas de Tinga and Tacos Vegetales. The latter came with small flour tortillas with zucchini that was tender but still had a nice bite and crunchiness, sautéed mushrooms, sweet bursts of corn, garlic, the perfect amount of heat from rajas poblanas, and earthy goat cheese. Each taco was two or three bites and despite being very messy, the tacos offered a blend of flavors and textures that will wake up your palate. The highlight of the dinner for me was the Tostadas de Tinga—lightly spiced chicken topped with roasted tomatoes, chipotle peppers, refried black beans, green tomatillo salsa, queso fresco, and sour cream. All of these flavors meld together, taking your taste buds on a journey of salty, sweet, and spice.

The tostada is freshly fried and the beans and roasted tomatoes burst in your mouth. It ends with a crunch that is contrasted by the creamy cheese and fresh sour cream on the top.

Day 3, and A, D, H, J, Q, T and Z are checked off the list. Lesson learned: visiting a restaurant with ethnic cuisine like San Angel can help hit the tough letters and get your teenager to try something new.

Day 4: Saturday

DISH 1. Popcorn, at a stand near Grauman's Chinese Theatre in Hollywood Studios. Popcorn is a staple at Disney theme parks. On this particular day, Austin and I were stopping for a salty treat near the Star Wars Launch Bay. Just as I shoveled a handful into my mouth, I turned right into the chest of a very large Stormtrooper. "Are you part of the First Order?" he demanded. Startled and feeling a bit "on the spot" with my Star Wars trivia, I swallowed and replied, "No?" The Stormtrooper looked at the two others with him and replied, "Are you sure you are not part of the First Order?" Remembering that the First Order is the bad guys and Chewy is my favorite Star Wars character, I replied more confidently, "No." The lead guy looked at his fellow troopers and asked, "Should we take her?" I said, emphatically: "No!" They looked at each other and then kept marching. Wonder what would have happened if I had said "yes" to that last question? Even boring old salty popcorn at Disney can be an enchanting experience.

DISH 2. The Sampling of Mom's Favorite Dishes (yep, that's the actual name on the menu!) at 50's Prime-Time Diner in Hollywood Studios. Prime Time is all about the experience. The food is just okay comfort food, like fried chicken, meatloaf, and mashed potatoes. The waitresses act as if they're busy, tired 1950s housewives or househusbands (were there any of those in the 1950s?). They're often impatient and tell funny jokes. At the end of our meal, the waitress came over to Austin and said, "Sweetie, I'm tired and had a long day, will you clear the table and get the dishes?" At first Austin hesitated, thinking she was kidding. The look on her face made it clear she was not. Austin obediently grabbed the dishes. "Follow me and we'll get these washed," the waitress said. About three minutes later he returned with an amused look on his face and said she had him take the dishes back into the kitchen, but then told him he was excused and could return to the table. At this point the entire room was looking at Austin and having a laugh at his interaction with our busy waitress. She got an extra generous tip for putting my teen to work.

I wonder if I was hungry at the end of Day 4? Only P and S were checked off the list. Stormtroopers harassed me and Austin had to do the dishes, so all in all, it was a pretty bizarre day of Disney dining.

Day 4.5: Sunday

DISH 1. Gingerbread cookie at Coronado Springs. Dotted throughout the parks and resorts are different holiday goodies, testing your (and your airline's) ability to safely transport fragile packages. One of those is a build-your-own gingerbread house, available at most gift shops. The kit includes the gingerbread, frosting, and brightly colored Mickey-shaped candies to adorn the festive house. It's a tempting display and someone had already pecked off one of the little Mickey candies. As tempting as it was to get G checked off the list and have a quick taste, I decided to have a gingerbread cookie that was right under the gingerbread house display. It tasted a bit mass-produced and the icing was so thick the entire thing just tasted of icing sugar. If you're going to do cookies at Disney, it's worth stopping at one of the many bakeries and having something fresh.

DISH 2. Naan and umami at Sanaa in Kidani Village at Animal Kingdom Lodge. During our trip in 2015 we visited Sanaa twice and Austin had been dreaming about the butter chicken ever since. Like mushrooms and bacon, butter chicken is an umami taste-sensation food. Austin and I both ordered the butter chicken and naan, very excited to have it once again.

Day 4.5 is over, G, N, and U are off the list, and sadly we were on the airplane home to bitterly cold and snowy Chicago.

Phew! That's a lot of food in 4 days and it was totally worth it. Would I do it again? Absolutely. Except I would have a bit more time and go to more resorts and definitely get a Zebra Dome from Animal Kingdom Lodge as my letter Z. Also, I'd do it with friends. Disney is home of the generous portions and the more people with you the more dishes you can try.

See pictures of all the foods from this Disney Dining Challenge. Just search on #DisneyEatsFromAtoZ.

APPENDIX C

Best of Disney Dining Lists

With over 300 places to eat, dining at Disney can either be an array of delicious choices or daunting and completely overwhelming. Need to know where to go? We've got you covered.

7 Restaurants You Won't Forget

- Be Our Guest at Magic Kingdom. As Chef Lee says, "You will hear it everywhere and it's 100% true, if you can get in, go to Be Our Guest. Even chefs will tell you, go in for the desserts. The desserts are beautiful. They're delicious. You will hear that from everyone, including pastry chefs. Disney has put a ton of their magic into those desserts."
- Cinderella's Royal Table at Magic Kingdom.
- Sci-Fi Dine-In Theater at Hollywood Studios.
- 50's Prime Time Café at Hollywood Studios. Eat dinner around the TV just like in the 1950s and see footage of opening day at Disneyland.
- Restaurant Marrakesh at Epcot. Belly dancers, live music, and beef with cinnamon and nutmeg.
- Whispering Canyon Café at Wilderness Lodge. If celebrating a birthday at Disney World, this is a fun place to go. They bring you a cupcake and make a lot of noise.
- Tiffins at Animal Kingdom.

3 Places Grandma & Grandpa Recommend

- Coral Reef Restaurant at Epcot. Grandma says, "Watching the fish is relaxing." Grandpa said, "I felt bad enjoying this delectable salmon while watching fish swim by." The view did not change how good he thought the food was.
- The BOATHOUSE at Disney Springs. Grandma says, "The food was unbelievable. We had the salmon on a cedar plank and have been planking it at home ever since."
- Pepper Market at Coronado Springs. So many options and choices. Grandpa says, "Fruit and yogurt every day and you can sit outside right on the water and watch the turtles."

5 Places Teens Will Love

- Starbucks anywhere. Teens love Starbucks.
- Be Our Guest at Magic Kingdom. It's really like being in a movie set from their childhood.
- Sci-Fi Dine-In Theatre at Hollywood Studios. It's like a drive-in movie theatre, though Austin pointed out, "Would be much better if you were there on a date. It's not as fun when you're sitting next to your mom."
- Ghirardelli in Disney Springs. Austin says, "The Sea Salt Caramel Chocolate Shake is insane. It's like Starbucks but even better!"
- Happy Landing Ice Cream at Typhoon Lagoon. Cast member Nick says, "They literally serve a bucket of ice cream. There's waffle cone, caramel syrup, chocolate syrup, strawberry syrup, cherries, they put all that in and then put ice cream on top. It's a sand bucket filled with ice cream."

5 Restaurants for Romance

- Les Chefs de France at Epcot. Sitting in the back sunroom in the evening and drinking French champagne with the glow from the fountain is a recipe for romance.
- San Angel Inn at Epcot.
- Tutto Gusto Wine Cellar at Epcot. Grab a small couch for two in front of the fireplace with a bottle of wine and be transported to a small Italian village.
- Victoria & Albert's at Grand Floridian.
- Paddlefish at Disney Springs. Visit Paddlefish at night and claim a comfy couch on the upper deck. This place has an expansive view of all of Disney Springs with plush seating, a full-service bar, and strings of dimly lit bulbs.

4 Loud Restaurants

- Crystal Palace at Magic Kingdom. This is a character meal and character meals have more kids and are pretty loud.
- Kona Café at the Polynesian Village.
- Whispering Canyon Café at Wilderness Lodge. You can hear the whooping and hollering coming from the restaurant before you can even see it.
- 50's Prime-Time Café at Hollywood Studios.

6 Places to Escape the Crowds

- Be Our Guest at Magic Kingdom, in the Castle Gallery room. Everyone wants to either sit in the main ballroom to feel as if they are Belle and Beast dancing the night away or in the dimly lit West Wing to watch the rose petals fall. The Castle Gallery is a bit tucked away to the right off the ballroom.

- Colombia Harbour House in Magic Kingdom. The booths have high backs and are tucked into corners. Try to get one of those or try the second level, which is a bit less busy.
- Restaurant Marrakesh in the Morocco Pavilion at Epcot. This restaurant is tucked far back in the pavilion. Even walking to it is quiet and relaxing with the gentle lull of the fountains and soft chatter of the locals.
- Sci-Fi Dine-In at Hollywood Studios can actually be an escape, if you are able to sit in a vehicle. The room is dark and cool and the movies are not very loud.
- Harambe Market at Animal Kingdom. The market is a bit off the beaten path with different seating areas, some covered and others tucked in corners.
- Tutto Gusto Wine Cellar at Epcot is always on our list of places to stop and cool off. It's a bit hidden away and easy to overlook, and rarely busy, despite its refreshing cocktails, low lighting, and comfy couches.

5 Magical Locations to Eat Gluten-Free

- Jiko at Animal Kingdom Lodge. Maggie says, "I didn't really think of it as gluten-free because I just had meat."
- Coral Reef at Epcot.
- Sanaa in Kidani Village at Animal Kingdom Lodge. Maggie says, "Disney magic has made it so I can have gluten-free Naan."
- Epcot International Flower & Garden Festival and Food & Wine Festival. In 2016 Maggie, our gluten-free expert, tried the grilled sweet and spicy bushberry shrimp with pineapple, pepper, onion, and snap peas at the Australia Marketplace and said that it "made gluten-free Disney a little more magical." Many marketplaces that offer gluten-free dishes. In the passport brochure, look for GF (gluten-free) or V (vegetarian) next to the item description.

Gluten-free Tip: Disney understands that guests have different dietary needs. At most table-service restaurants there is a gluten-free specific menu and some quick-service locations also offer an allergy menu. Ask a cast member for a menu or for special dietary accommodations if you need them. The best festival to be gluten-free is Food & Wine with its over ten different GF items on offer at the various marketplaces. Flower & Garden comes in second with seven in 2017, but gets a bonus point for a GF dessert called macaron chocolate framboise.

6 Places for the True Disney Foodies

- Jiko at Animal Kingdom Lodge. Jiko is in the top restaurant for gourmet dining in all of Disney World. You will have to have traveled to some pretty exotic locales if you don't find something you haven't tried on the menu here.
- Tiffins at Animal Kingdom is the newest gourmet restaurant in a park and is a culinary journey for all of your senses. From the incredible architecture and the three distinct dining rooms, to a menu where each dish and drink has a story, Tiffins will transport you to another world.
- Victoria & Albert's at the Grand Floridian Resort. Sam says, "There was a stool just for my purse!"
- California Grill at the Contemporary Resort. Chef Vance from Coronado Springs says, "California Grill must be on your list. Whenever I have family or friends in town and we want an amazing experience, we go to California Grill."
- Drinks Around the World/Epcot Pub Crawl. Cast member Nicoletta from Tutto Gusto Wine Cellar says, "You have margaritas in Mexico, a beer in Germany, and come to Tutto Gusto for a nice cocktail with Prosecco or Italian wine." Chef Lee says, "Because foodies drink, you must

try Epcot doing the Drinks Around the World. Start early. Have a friend. Share the experience. Probably best to share the drinks so you can make it through. Eleven countries is a lot of booze."

- Epcot International Food & Wine Festival. Chef Bruno says,"My favorite bite at Disney was at Food & Wine. There is food that I love." When it comes to food, always listen to a French chef! Chef Lee agrees: "If you can make it to Food & Wine, that is insane. It's new every year. Trying to make it through the passport and check everything off is a must-do. You want to be a true foodie, you have to do Food & Wine."

Acknowledgments

Thank you for adding this book to your Disney library. Writing about Disney is magical—almost as magical as eating at Disney!

For all those folks out there that read my first book, *The Not-So-Evil Stepmother in the Most Magical Place on Earth*, thank you. It was your support that gave me the confidence to write this book. Connecting with fellow Disney fans is one of the best parts about writing about Disney. Find me on Facebook @authorTrishaDaab or Instagram @notsoevil_disneystepmom. If you're struggling with where to dine, please contact me. I love helping folks find their Disney food magic.

To all who have come to this happy place called Disney and are cast members, thank you. It is your smiles, your passion, and your commitment to the magic that makes a Disney vacation a vacation like no other.

To all the cast members and Disney chefs that have raised the bar on what food at a theme park can and should be, my stomach and I thank you.

Thank you to the supportive community of Disney fans on Instagram. You are a constant source of smiles and ideas, and are the perfect quick Disney fix. Special thanks to:

@summerlovesdisney
@_followthemagic
@_mama3curlies
@adventures.with.carissa
@belixoxo27
@chaos_and_couture
@christinessmess
@crazyholley
@hayleescomett
@kaylee.kwaytaal
@main_st_brown

@mais_oui_disney
@mar_shurt
@pnwdisneylover
@rachiedawns
@the_little_tsum
@theselfishunicorn
@themainstreetmoms
@tt_choppa
@wishesdishes_wdwdelights

The Disney Dining Challenge: Disney Eats from A-Z would not have been possible without all of your ideas.

To the six amazing cast members who shared your passion and love of Disney food for this book, thank you.

Chef Bruno, thank you for giving up your lunch break to share your incredible Disney history and story. Chef Vance, it was meeting you on that Disney transport bus that triggered the idea of including cast members in this book. Thank you for the inspiration. Chef Lee, thank you for the multiple very long but incredibly amusing phone calls. You always make me smile. Nicoletta, your passion for Disney and Italy is infectious. And your story about your Papa and chicken parmigiana will definitely be in my next book about Disney food. Nick, you spent so much time and gave up more than one evening to answer my long list of questions. You have a knack for storytelling and have so many amazing Disney memories. I am honored you let me share them in this book. Mallorie, you have solidified Les Chefs de France as one of our favorite places at Disney World. You are just like elegant French champagne—effervescent.

Jamie, my short girl, boozy, water-loving compadre. Thank you for all the late night text marathons, for being a Disney expert editor, for jumping into the podcast deep end with me, and for being amazing wonderful funny you. Someday we will go to Disney to eat all the food and get the meat sweats.

Bob McLain of Theme Park Press took a chance on *Not-So-Evil Stepmother*, my first book. Thank you, Bob, for putting up with all my questions and emails, and for supporting a different kind of guide to Disney food.

To all our friends who read my first book, wrote reviews, came to book signings, and dominated Disney pub trivia, thank you. Nick, aka Nickolas. Thanks for letting me call you Nickolas and for being willing to try new foods and answer all my questions with a smile.

Samantha Daab is an incredibly talented artist. Thank you so much for working with me again and for making Disney food look even cooler. We are so, so proud you are a Daab.

To Nate, Mags, Annie, Austin, and Oliver. You are always willing to try new things and then put up with me grilling you about it later. You are all kind, creative, and always make me smile. I am so proud to have you call me Mom/Mama/Stepmom/Trish.

Last, to my best food-loving friend and husband, Joe. Thank you for patiently waiting for me to take pictures of every single dish before you could take a bite. And for being all proud and telling everyone we met at Disney that I wrote a book. Everything just tastes better when we are experiencing it together.

About the Author

Trisha Daab is an author, mom/not-so-evil stepmom, marketing strategist, and food lover. She is the author of *The Not-So-Evil Stepmother in the Most Magical Place on Earth: Planning Your Walt Disney World Family Vacation* and is the co-host of a Disney food segment on the DizRadio podcast. According to her sons and husband, she takes way too many pictures at Disney.

Trisha has been visiting Disney since she her first trip at 3 years old in the 80s. She even has a *very* embarrassing picture with Chewbacca in all of her coke-bottle-glasses-and-90s-hair glory. Writing books about Disney World has been the perfect excuse to visit the parks more frequently, eat a lot of Disney food, and get new pictures with Chewy.

You can find out more about her, get updates on her next book, check out pics from the Disney food challenge, and see that epic 90s hair on Instagram @notsoevil_disneystepmom and on Facebook @authorTrishaDaab.

ABOUT THEME PARK PRESS

Theme Park Press publishes books primarily about the Disney company, its history, culture, films, animation, and theme parks, as well as theme parks in general.

Our authors include noted historians, animators, Imagineers, and experts in the theme park industry.

We also publish many books by first-time authors, with topics ranging from fiction to theme park guides.

And we're always looking for new talent. If you'd like to write for us, or if you're interested in the many other titles in our catalog, please visit:

www.ThemeParkPress.com

Theme Park Press Newsletter

Subscribe to our free email newsletter and enjoy:

- Free book downloads and giveaways
- Access to excerpts from our many books
- Announcements of forthcoming releases
- Exclusive additional content and chapters
- And more good stuff available nowhere else

To subscribe, visit www.ThemeParkPress.com, or send email to newsletter@themeparkpress.com.

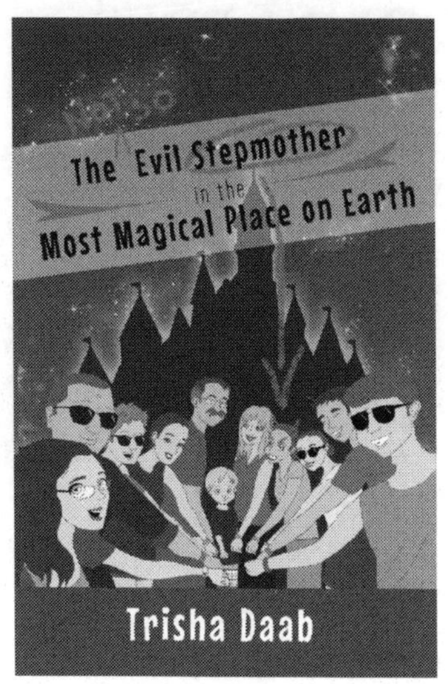
The Evil Stepmother
in the
Most Magical Place on Earth
Trisha Daab

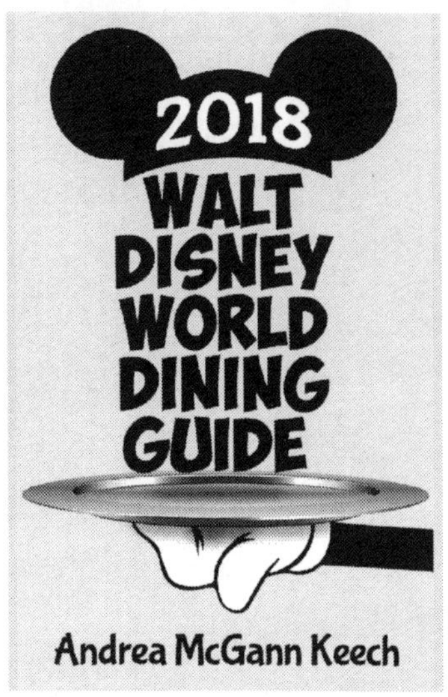
2018
WALT
DISNEY
WORLD
DINING
GUIDE
Andrea McGann Keech

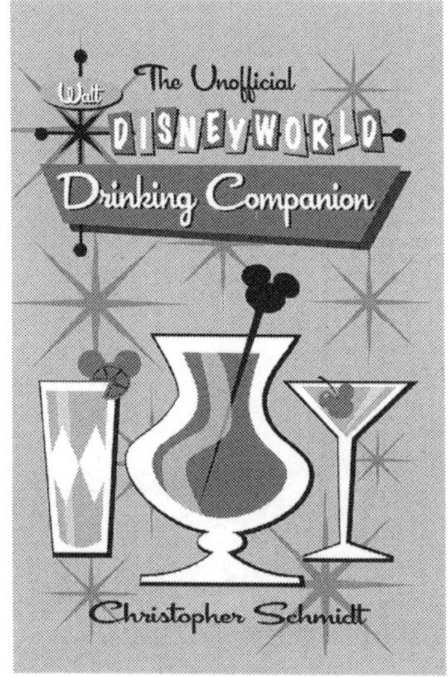
The Unofficial
Walt
DISNEYWORLD
Drinking Companion
Christopher Schmidt

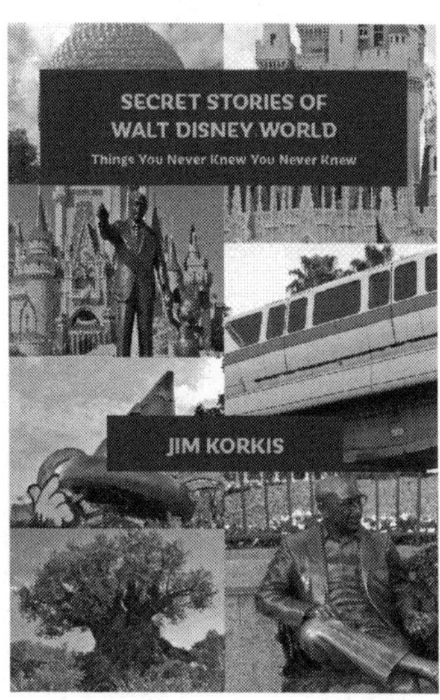
SECRET STORIES OF
WALT DISNEY WORLD
Things You Never Knew You Never Knew
JIM KORKIS

Made in the USA
San Bernardino, CA
11 April 2018